Michael van Straten

super
energy

detox

quadrille

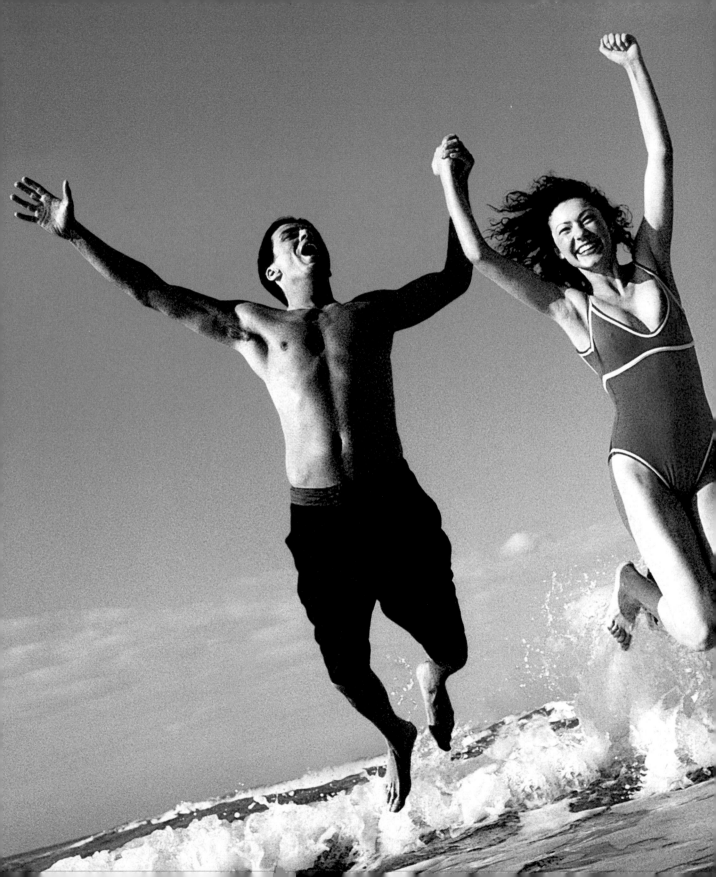

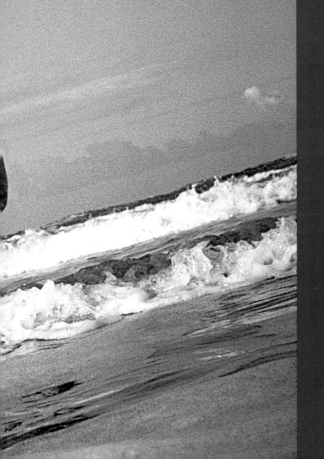

contents

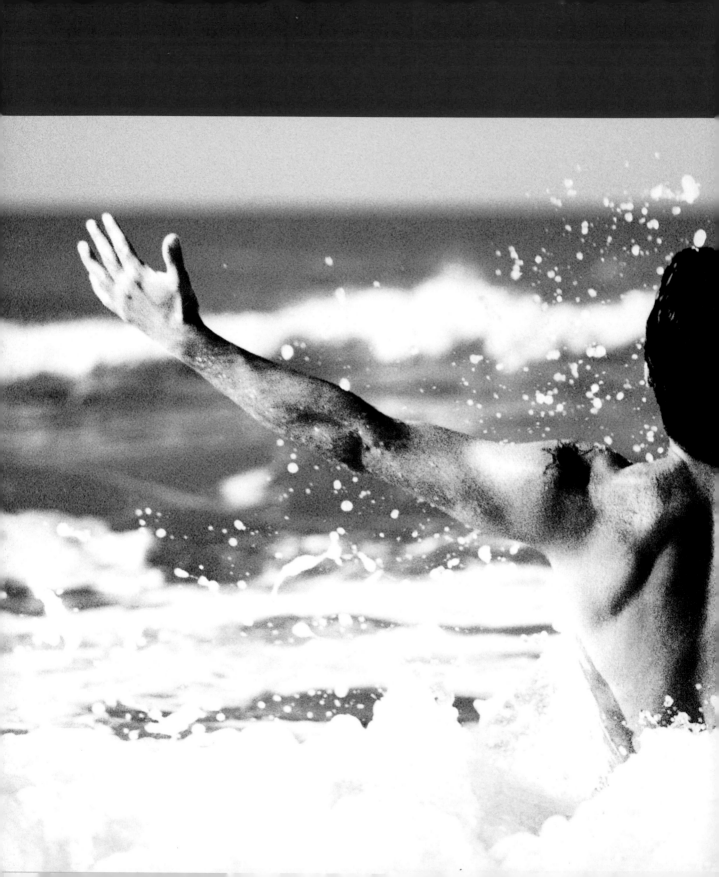

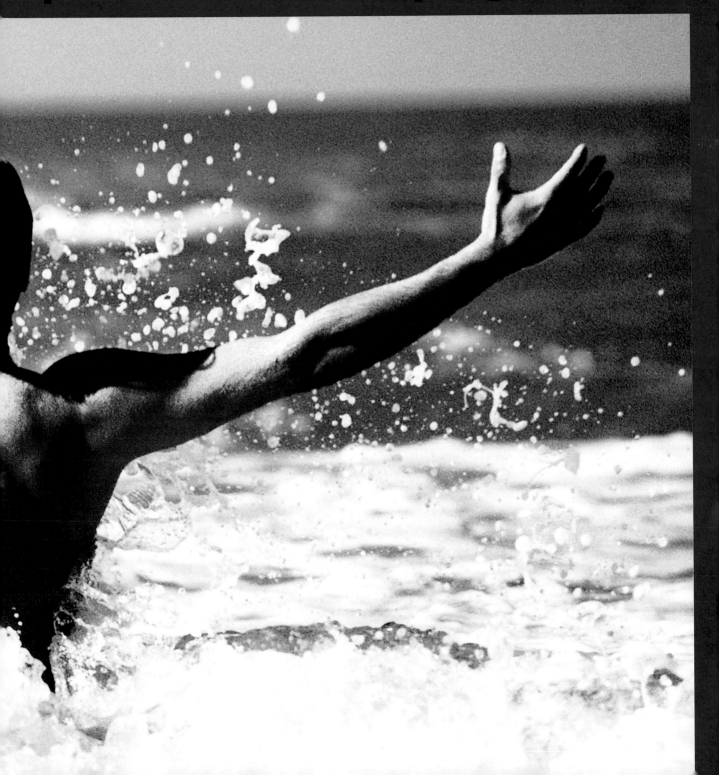

the search for super energy

Energy is the key to life, whether you think of it as a spiritual energy, a flowing life force like the 'chi' of Chinese medicine, or the electrical impulses that scientists tell us govern every bodily function. Without an adequate supply of mental, spiritual and physical energy, leading a full life becomes impossible and maintaining good health is out of the question.

Energy equates with vitality and we all know people whose boundless and unquenchable vitality seems to have no limits. These are the people who are the 'doers', the creators, the rocks in an emergency, the steadfast friends in a crisis. But their performance is not built just on their goodwill, kindness or humanity. Without the energy to follow through, their good intentions would fall at the first hurdle.

But millions of you wake up every morning feeling exhausted and worn out. In fact, tiredness is one of the most common problems that send you to your doctor. Overheated, stuffy buildings and crowded public transport take their toll. Who knows what else you catch when you catch your morning train? Traffic jams and bad weather turn even the most mild mannered into road-rage maniacs. And the depressing thought of another routine day in a frustrating job that you don't enjoy, the stresses of dealing with the public or a demanding, insensitive boss are enough to make you go straight back to bed and hide under the duvet.

Working mums often have a lot of extra pressures to cope with on top of all this, and if these weren't enough on its own, when winter brings short days, lack of sunlight and Seasonal Affective Disorder (SAD), the agony just gets piled on.

In an ideal world we would all be living on a carefully balanced diet that keeps the baddies to a minimum and is chock-full of nutritious ingredients. Sadly, we're so busy that few of us have the time or the energy to plan our shopping and eating in advance. In addition, for many young mothers, life is a permanent battle with difficult children who want to exist on nothing but fish fingers and instant desserts. And how many of you have husbands or boyfriends who think they'll die of malnutrition if they don't have meat at least twice a day?

Don't turn to the bottle and don't take tranquillisers, but most certainly, don't give up. All you need is Super Energy Detox. You'll be amazed at how quickly it will give you that surge of extra energy, an all-over glow of well-being and a feeling of immense relief as the weight lifts from your shoulders and you return once again to being a fully functioning human being. Renewing your vital forces will help your body to overcome disease and damage, and your mind to deal with its problems. In fact, Super Energy Detox will help maintain both your physical and spiritual well-being in the state that is your birthright.

my top twelve energy superfoods

Nature has provided us with a powerhouse of energy-giving foods, so when you're dashing around the supermarket or snatching a quick lunch break, do yourself a favour – avoid those high-fat, high-sugar fast foods and swap them for my top 12 energy superfoods.

1 baked potatoes
Rich in fibre, vitamins B and C, potassium and with no fat. Don't add mayonnaise, butter or cream cheese but serve with spicy tomato sauce and green salad.

2 pasta
Instant energy that will also keep you going for three or four hours. Add tuna, tomato sauce, stir-fried vegetables or, as millions of Italians do every day, a drizzle of olive oil and some finely chopped garlic. Go easy on the Parmesan.

3 beans
Good old baked beans, like all their relatives, provide slow-release energy and are rich in protein, carbohydrates and soluble fibre. Tinned beans are fine, but rinse well to remove the salt. Use in salads, soups, and casseroles for a real vitality boost.

4 rice
Very low in fat, with protein, B vitamins and, especially if it's brown, masses of slow-release energy. Brown rice takes a little longer to cook but provides more of all the nutrients. Eat it hot for your evening meal and take the leftovers to work in a rice salad.

5 bananas
Nature's miracle fast food. They're not fattening and are full of essential nutrients like potassium, zinc, iron, vitamin B6 and folic acid, as well as instant energy. They're easily digested and their high potassium content helps prevent cramp.

6 sweetcorn
Seldom on the list of healthy foods, but one of my favourites and a great energy booster. Add to salads and soups, or eat with a modest amount of butter and lots of black pepper.

7 fruit

All fruit, including dried, is a source of instant energy. Their natural sugars are quickly digested to give an instant power boost.

8 oats

The cheapest and best breakfast of all, offering B vitamins for your nervous system, vitamin E for your heart and skin, and slow-release energy which will keep you going till lunchtime without the mid-morning munchies. Start the day with porridge or muesli.

9 nuts and seeds

Not chocolate-covered, not salted, just natural. Delicious and rich in protein and minerals, particularly zinc and selenium. Not for instant energy but offering a gentle continual energy release, which makes them perfect to carry around and nibble on during the day.

10 buckwheat

You may never have heard of it and probably haven't knowingly tasted it, but it makes those wonderful French, Dutch and Belgian pancakes as well as the ones served with Chinese duck. Not a cereal, but a relative of rhubarb, as well as providing loads of energy, it's great for the circulation and helps reduce high blood pressure.

11 lentils

Very high in protein and contain lots of iron to prevent anaemia and stop you feeling tired. They also contain B vitamins for memory and mental faculties and are a great source of fat-free, energy-giving calories. Delicious in traditional Indian dhal or on their own with meat dishes or in salads.

12 bread

The staff of life, but because people think it's fattening, we don't eat nearly enough. Wholemeal is of course best, but there are now so many wonderful breads available that you can mix and match in any way you like to get at least four or five slices a day. Bread contains masses of energy, virtually no fat – unless you smother it with butter – lots of B vitamins and everything you need to keep you on the go. Never eat slimming bread, low-calorie bread, or the cheap sliced white bread that's like cotton wool.

my top five energy superherbs

When you're eating my top twelve energy superfoods, don't forget that natural herbs can help your energy levels too. Add them to your cooking for a double dose of energy. You can never have too much.

1 rosemary

This versatile herb is a rich source of volatile essential oils and flavonoids which are extremely energising as well as mood-enhancing. It also boosts your brain power and memory. It is perfect in soups, salads and pasta dishes and is ideal for flavouring oils, vinegars and marinades.

2 sage

This gives a real power boost to your energy levels, but only if you use the right variety. The most important constituent for energy is the natural substance thujone, but there's virtually none of that in the commonly sold Spanish sage. For the richest source and most potent energy booster, use purple sage, which is particularly good for women as it helps even out those hormone imbalances that are the cause of low energy levels. Add sage to almost any savoury dish you like or use it to make a tea.

3 marjoram

This is the ideal energizing herb to accompany oily fish, casseroles or meat dishes. It contains anti-viral and anti-bacterial eugenol and energy-boosting estragole. Often called sweet marjoram, it's the most potent of this family of plants and is closely related to oregano, hence its botanical name, **Oreganum majorana**.

4 lavender

Everyone knows that lavender oil is good for headaches, but few people make use of this wonderful herb in cooking. It contains more than 40 plant chemicals, with masses of energy-boosting volatile oils, protective coumarins and flavonoids. Use the flowers to make a delicious and refreshing tea, add them to biscuits, cakes or ice creams or, surprisingly, use them together with the finely chopped leaves in rich meat-based soups, casseroles and stews.

5 bay

This is a rather abused herb which is often overlooked for its valuable medicinal properties. A rich source of energizing laurenolide, bay is also good for chest infections and depression as well as bringing on delayed periods.

In addition to the traditional use in savoury dishes, try it in all milk-based puddings as it enhances their flavours in a surprising way. It really is worth growing your own as the fresh leaves have a much more subtle and delicate taste than the dried.

why fast?

But first you really must fast. I know it seems like the last thing you want to do if your energy levels are at rock bottom, but fasting is Nature's great energizer and rejuvenator. It also helps deal with long-term chronic illness – another common cause of serious energy deficiency. It does this by making the body more efficient at destroying invading organisms and so increasing your natural resistance to infection. Fasting also encourages the body to heal its damaged tissues and, most importantly of all, it encourages homoeostasis – the mechanism that maintains the body's chemical stability, without which we couldn't survive.

My detoxing for energy programmes are, of necessity, quite drastic and rigid to begin with, but amazing results will follow if you stick to the advice. If you have any underlying health problems or if your severe lack of energy can't be attributed to an obvious cause, you should seek your doctor's advice before embarking on these regimes.

time to detox?

Zest, pzazz, charisma, fit, 'it', buzz, aura – all wonderful words that really mean energy. Are you blessed with it or do you constantly feel that your get up and go has got up and gone? Even if you think you've never had it, I can assure you that you can have it, and sooner than you think thanks to Super Energy Detox. To find out if you're an energy giant, and if not why not, answer these simple questions.

1 What do you do first thing in the morning?
- **A** I get up when I wake up.
- **B** I snooze for 10 minutes then get up.
- **C** I go back to sleep and wake up an hour later feeling dreadful.

2 How many hours sleep do you get a night?
- **A** 5 or 6.
- **B** less than 5.
- **C** more than 8.

3 Are you a snorer?
- **A** Not as far as I know.
- **B** Only if I have a cold or drink too much.
- **C** The neighbours bang on the wall most nights.

4 Do you take sleeping pills?
- **A** Never.
- **B** Rarely.
- **C** Every night.

5 How many cups of tea and coffee do you drink each day?
- **A** 4 or less without sugar.
- **B** 4–8 without sugar.
- **C** More than 8 without sugar (if you take sugar add 2 points per cup to your final score).

6 What is the total weight of sweets and chocolates you eat each day?
- **A** 100g or less.
- **B** 100–200g.
- **C** more than 200g.

7 Do you (tick as many as you like)
Smoke?
Drink more than 14 units (women) or 21 units (men) of alcohol a week?
Take tranquillisers or antidepressants?
Use recreational drugs?

8 Which of the following sums up your exercise pattern?
- **A** No problems on that score. I'm at the gym most nights of the week.
- **B** I don't do much, but I probably get half an hour's exercise three or four times a week.
- **C** I don't do any if I can possibly avoid it.

9 How much time do you spend on your favourite hobby?
- **A** At least 4 hours a week.
- **B** Less than 4 hours a week.
- **C** I don't have time for hobbies.

10 When you come home from work, sit in the armchair and watch your favourite soap on TV, do you fall asleep in the middle?

    A Never.

    B Occasionally.

    C Nearly always.

11 Do you nod off at inappropriate moments, for example in the middle of dinner, at your office desk, during a work meeting, in the cinema or theatre?

    A No.

    B Very rarely.

    C Embarrassingly often.

12 Do you feel exhausted most of the time?

    A No.

    B Only at the end of a long hard week.

    C All the time, even when I wake up in the morning.

13 Do you have chronic digestive problems like indigestion, irritable bowel syndrome, bloating or wind?

    A Not at all.

    B Occasionally if I eat things which I know don't agree with me.

    C Yes, after almost every meal.

14 Do you eat regular meals on most days?

    A Usually, but it's not always possible.

    B Not very often as I'm too tired to bother when I get home.

    C Hardly ever. I don't have time for breakfast. I eat nibbles during the day and maybe have a takeaway in the evening.

15 If somebody suggested you had a stressful life, what would you say?

    A Stressful? Never heard of the word.

    B Well, isn't everybody occasionally?

    C I haven't got time to answer that question – look at all the work I have to do.

Score:

    A – 1 point

    B – 3 points

    C or tick – 5 points

Over 85 – your energy levels are at an all-time low and you're going to have to make a supreme effort just to get to the shops to buy the ingredients for the energy detox that you need so urgently. You'll be amazed by the surge of energy you'll feel afterwards. It'll give you the ability to make the serious changes to your lifestyle and diet – for instance including regular amounts of all my recommended energy superfoods – that you need for a long-term solution to your lack of energy.

60–85 – you probably feel okay sometimes but when things pile up, your eating gets worse and you soon burn off your energy reserves and start to find life a struggle. Once you've tried energy detoxing, you'll see that you can even out these ups and downs and restore some balance to your life.

35–60 – you're the one who will have the energy and vitality to take on the challenge of detoxing right now, even though you need it least. Use the plans in this book and incorporate plenty of my recommended energy-rich foods, and everyone else will still have problems keeping up with you when you're in your eighties.

Under 35 – I'm glad I don't live with you. You're probably up at dawn and still clubbing at midnight. You've got boundless energy but I suspect there may be a bit too much. There is, after all, a difference between being super-energetic and hyperactive. Calm down a little and make some time to stand and stare.

cleansing for

If you're suffering from real exhaustion and chronic fatigue, you've just got to take the bull by the horns and follow my full three-day Cleansing for Energy detox followed by the eight-day return to normal eating.

For patients of mine who have struggled with a lack of energy for years, I advise that they aim to do this combination of programmes four times a year. Once they've tried it they've found – as I'm sure you will too – that the benefits are so obvious and their energy has received such an enormous boost, that they're happy to stick to this pattern. And it's always a lot easier the second time around.

While you're following the programmes, it's really important to take my advice on the supplements you need (see pages 16–17), and before you start, don't forget to check with your doctor to make sure the programmes are suitable for you. If your lack of energy is not due to some serious underlying illness, there are few contra-indications.

energy

short of time?

If it's difficult to take a few days off – which you really need if you're going to do the full programme – then follow the twenty-four hour detox once a week or the forty-eight hour programme once a month. You'll soon notice an increase in your general energy and vitality.

And as a bonus, these Cleansing for Energy plans will boost your natural resistance to disease, significantly lower your blood pressure and cholesterol levels, improve your liver function and help make you mentally more positive and alert.

side effects

You'll feel some side effects when you're fasting, even on a twenty-four hour programme. The most common side effect is a headache, caused by the drop in your blood-sugar levels and by the fact that your body is starting to eliminate its accumulation of waste. Try not to take painkillers as the headache will soon pass. Drinking plenty of water will help.

the extras

My Cleansing for Energy plans are quite drastic and your body will need extra support to help it through. Even the eight-day return to normal eating regime is based on a fairly limited food intake, and although it does include a lot of high-nutrient foods, you'll need some extra support for this too.

There are three groups of supplements you need to take each day to help you on any of the programmes.

supportive supplements to maintain nutrient levels

▶ 1 high potency multi-vitamin and mineral supplement (choose one of the reputable brand leaders)

▶ 500mg vitamin C, three times a day. If possible, take ester-C as it's non-acidic and less likely to cause digestive upsets, especially while you're on a restricted diet

▶ A high-potency B-complex to nourish the central nervous system and stimulate energy conversion

supplements that help the body convert food into available energy

▶ Co-enzyme Q – a powerful antioxidant and especially valuable for chronic fatigue, glandular fever, tired-all-the-time syndrome and ME

▶ Kelp – a major source of iodine. This controls the thyroid gland, which is vital for the production of energy

supplements that directly increase the body's energy supply

▶ Guarana – the extraordinary herb used as a source of energy by the Indians of the Brazilian rainforest for more than a thousand years. It's unique in its ability to produce gradual slow-release, long-term energy, rather than the quick boost and let-down that you get from a cup of strong coffee or a can of cola.

▶ Ginseng – used by the Chinese as an energy medicine for more than six thousand years. It not only boosts physical and mental energy, but as a bonus helps increase natural immunity and the body's ability to resist the damaging effects of stress.

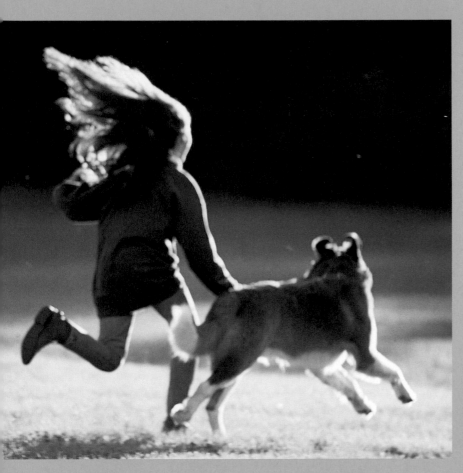

rest and relaxation

People are incredulous when I say that a combination of fasting and gentle exercise will help improve their energy levels – until they try it themselves. By giving your body a rest from high-fat, high-sugar foods, you'll find you can generate much more sustainable energy.

Detoxing does put some strain on your physical resources though, so it's essential to get enough rest while you're doing it. But there's a delicate balance to be struck. Having a lie-in in the morning is fine, so is putting your feet up for 10 minutes a few times a day. But your body needs to be active. This will not only stimulate your heart, circulation and breathing, and get your liver working, but it will trigger the release of the activity hormones that you're so obviously lacking.

And don't overdo the physical exertion, in the belief that you'll be detoxing more effectively. You won't. Your body will just be producing toxic chemical by-products, which will defeat the whole object of detoxing. You'll also be draining your energy reserves. Two or three 15-minute walks a day are ideal. Jogging or going to the gym aren't.

what to drink

While you're detoxing you need to keep up your fluid intake. I always recommend drinking as much filtered water, low-mineral-content bottled water or herb tea as you like, but not adding milk or sweetener. And canned drinks, squashes, fizzy water, cordials, Indian tea, coffee, and alcohol are definite no-nos, as are sugar-free commercial drinks since these contain artificial sweeteners.

twenty-four hour cleansing

The day before your twenty-four hour energy detox, avoid all animal protein and have a fairly light diet of just fruit, vegetables and salads. Drink at least one and a half litres of water and reduce your caffeine intake to lessen the likelihood of headaches on the following day. At bedtime take a natural bulk laxative like psyllium seeds or linseeds. You can certainly follow this twenty-four hour plan while you're at work, but it's easier if you have a day at home.

on waking	A large glass of hot water with a thick slice of organic unwaxed lemon
breakfast	A large glass of hot water with a thick slice of organic unwaxed lemon A glass of unsweetened pineapple juice
mid-morning	A large glass of hot water with a thick slice of organic unwaxed lemon
lunch	A large glass of hot water with a thick slice of organic unwaxed lemon A large glass of any salt-free vegetable juice A mug of ginseng tea
mid-afternoon	A large glass of hot water with a thick slice of organic unwaxed lemon
supper	Mango, Kiwi and Pineapple Juice (see recipe, page 85) A mug of raspberry leaf tea
evening	A large glass of hot water with a thick slice of organic unwaxed lemon Carrot, Apple and Celery Juice (see recipe, page 85)
bedtime	A mug of camomile tea

forty-eight hour cleansing

Start by following the twenty-four hour Cleansing for Energy plan, then have:

on waking   A large glass of hot water with a thick slice of organic unwaxed lemon

breakfast   A large glass of hot water with a thick slice of organic unwaxed lemon and quarter of a teaspoon of powdered cinnamon – this tends to float on top of the water even if you stir
A large bunch of grapes
A mug of lemon and ginger tea

mid-morning   A large glass of hot water with a thick slice of organic unwaxed lemon

lunch   An apple, a stick of celery and 6 radishes
A large glass of tomato juice
A mug of mint tea

mid-afternoon   A large glass of hot water with a thick slice of organic unwaxed lemon

supper   A mango, 60g blueberries and a pear
4 ready-to-eat prunes
A glass of unsalted mixed vegetable juice

evening   A large glass of hot water with a thick slice of organic unwaxed lemon
Hauser Broth (see recipe, page 99)

bedtime   A mug of camomile tea with a teaspoon of organic honey

three-day cleansing

When it comes to boosting your energy levels, it really does pay to go straight into the three-day Cleansing for Energy detox plan if at all possible. When you wake up on the morning of day 4, you'll feel like a new person – full of vim and vigour and raring to get on with life. Be careful though. The temptation to do all those things you've been putting off for months must be resisted, otherwise you'll dissipate all the benefits that you've worked so hard for. Take things gently and ease yourself gradually back into your normal routine.

The three-day cleansing is serious detoxing and you really can't do it and continue with your usual work. You'll also need at least one rest day afterwards to allow your system to return to normal, so this is where a duvet day will come in handy.

As a naturopath, I've used this plan for my patients for almost 40 years and although it's not strictly speaking a complete fast, it's the nearest you can safely get to one without professional supervision. These three days are very low in calories but you will be surprised at how soon you stop feeling hungry. To help overcome the hunger pangs, take two teaspoons of the Swiss Herbal Tonic BioStrath Elixir, three times a day, and don't forget your supportive and energy-boosting supplements (see pages 16–17).

On days 1 and 2, follow the forty-eight hour Cleansing for Energy plan. Day 3 is an animal-protein- and dairy-product-free day that will optimise the energy-giving benefits of the first two days.

Days 1 and 2, follow the Forty-Eight Hour Cleansing programme. Day 3:

on waking
A large glass of hot water with a thick slice of organic unwaxed lemon

breakfast
A large glass of hot water with a thick slice of organic unwaxed lemon
Half a cantaloupe melon filled with fresh berries
A mug of rosehip tea

mid-morning
Carrot, Apple and Beetroot Juice (see recipe, page 84)

lunch
A large glass of hot water with a thick slice of organic unwaxed lemon
A bowl of Porridge with Cinnamon and Dried Fruits made with water (see recipe, page 80)
A large glass of tomato juice

mid-afternoon
A large glass of hot water with a thick slice of organic unwaxed lemon

supper
A large glass of hot water with a thick slice of organic unwaxed lemon
A mixture of chopped steamed leek, cabbage, spinach and kale, drizzled with olive oil
and lemon juice and with a generous sprinkling of nutmeg
A large glass of carrot juice
A mug of mint tea

evening
4 each dried or soaked prunes and apricots

bedtime
1 slice of wholemeal bread with a little honey
A mug of mint tea

eight-day return to normal eating

You really must try to follow this eight-day plan immediately after the three-day detox. Doing so will maximise your energy gain and help your digestive system return to normal in a measured and gradual way. If you're not able to follow the plan exactly, then for at least three days after the three-day detox, try to avoid all animal protein and dairy products, and stick to a diet of raw or cooked fruit, vegetables and salads, together with modest amounts of bread, potatoes, rice and pasta. You should then introduce small amounts of the other food groups gradually over the next two or three days.

While you're following the eight-day plan, you may swap whole days around, or eat your main meal at lunchtime and your light meal in the evening, if that suits you, but don't take one meal from one day and one from another as you could end up with an imbalance in your diet. It's also a good idea to take a teaspoon of the Swiss Herbal BioStrath Elixir three times a day for a bit of extra support.

drinking habits

Having got into the habit of drinking much more fluid than you were probably used to before, try to continue, as fluid improves the efficiency of your digestive system and the amount of essential nutrients that your body absorbs from your food. And as before, you should keep on drinking a minimum of one and a half litres a day of still mineral water, filtered tap water, or herb teas. And now that you've got used to starting your day with hot water and lemon, you should try and continue.

day 1

breakfast An orange, half a grapefruit, a large slice of melon
A glass of unsalted vegetable juice
A mug of herb tea

light meal A plateful of raw red and yellow peppers, cucumber, tomato, broccoli, cauliflower, celery, carrots, radishes and lots of fresh parsley, dressed with extra-virgin olive oil and lemon juice
A large glass of unsweetened fruit juice

main meal A large mixed salad of lettuce, tomato, watercress, onion, garlic, beetroot, celeriac, fresh mint and any herbs you like, with extra-virgin olive oil and lemon juice
A large glass of unsweetened fruit juice or unsalted vegetable juice

day 2

breakfast A bowl of Porridge with Cinnamon and Dried Fruits made with water (see recipe, page 80)
A large glass of Mango, Kiwi and Pineapple Juice (see recipe, page 85)

light meal Half an avocado, sliced, with watercress, tomatoes and cucumber, on mixed leaves with a generous squeeze of lemon juice
1 wholewheat roll
2 kiwi fruit
A large glass of unsalted vegetable juice

main meal A large bowl of Vegetable, Bean and Barley Soup (see recipe, page 98)
A large slice of melon and a bunch of grapes

day 3

breakfast Real Swiss Muesli (see recipe, page 80)
A glass of half-orange, half-grapefruit juice

light meal Papaya and Watercress Salad (see recipe, page 102)
1 slice of wholemeal bread and 2 tablespoons of Hummous (see recipe, page 102)
1 apple

main meal Spanish Omelette (see recipe, page 88) with mixed green salad
Spiced Baked Apple (see recipe, page 104)
A large glass of hot water with a thick slice of organic unwaxed lemon

day 4

It's vital for your system that you follow this 'rice' day exactly as it's laid out since it's an important part of your cleansing and energizing treatment. The most convenient way of going about it is to prepare the rice you need for the whole day, so start by cooking 100g dry-weight brown rice in half a litre of water, or 50g in water and the remaining 50g in vegetable stock for a more savoury flavour. In addition, make sure you drink at least an extra four large glasses of water during the day.

breakfast
85g cooked rice with 140g stewed apple flavoured with honey, cinnamon and grated lemon rind
A large glass of hot water with a thick slice of organic unwaxed lemon

mid-morning
A large glass of hot water with a thick slice of organic unwaxed lemon

lunch
85g cooked rice with 200g steamed vegetables – celery, leek, carrot, tomato, spinach, broccoli and shredded cabbage
A large glass of hot water with a thick slice of organic unwaxed lemon

mid-afternoon
A large glass of hot water with a thick slice of organic unwaxed lemon

supper
85g cooked rice mixed with soaked dried apricots, raisins and sultanas, and the flesh of a pink grapefruit
A large glass of hot water with a thick slice of organic unwaxed lemon

bedtime
A mug of camomile tea with a teaspoon of organic honey

day 5

breakfast
Half a pink grapefruit, baked beans (make sure you buy organic low-salt, low-sugar beans) on wholemeal toast with a large poached or grilled tomato

light meal
Italian Toast (see recipe, page 88)
Dried Fruit Compôte – make enough for 2 meals (see recipe, page 105)

main meal
Green Pasta with Tuna Fish (see recipe, page 86)
Half a pineapple with 2 tablespoons fromage frais and any fresh berries

day 6

breakfast   Dried Fruit Compôte (see recipe, page 105) with low-fat live yoghurt and an orange

light meal   Gratin of Potatoes – no they're not fattening! – and Mushrooms
(see recipe, page 89)
Glass of Carrot, Apple and Beetroot Juice (see recipe, page 84)

main meal   Cabbage Soup with Potatoes (see recipe, page 98)
Tuna and Mixed Bean Salad (see recipe, page 101)
An apple and a pear

day 7

breakfast   2 hot wholewheat rolls with a little butter
1 banana, a large glass of orange juice

light meal   A large portion of Red, White and Green Coleslaw (see recipe, page 100) with cottage cheese
1 peach or nectarine or 3 fresh apricots

main meal   Non-Meatballs in Tomato Sauce (see recipe, page 90) with pasta and Tomato and Red Onion Salad (see recipe, page 101)
Mango and Kiwi Sorbet (see recipe, page 104)

day 8

breakfast   Scrambled Eggs with Smoked Salmon (see recipe, page 81)
1 thin slice of wholemeal toast
Juice of a lemon in a large glass of water

light meal   Papaya and Watercress Salad (see recipe, page 102)
2 rye crispbreads with a matchbox-sized piece of Brie

main meal   Cold Beetroot and Apple Soup (see recipe, page 98)
Spiced Chickpea Casserole (see recipe, page 90)
Fresh fruit salad

cleansing summary

The Cleansing for Energy detox was really hard and extremely demanding, especially when you may have been suffering from chronic fatigue, exhaustion and an all-round lack of energy and enthusiasm when you started. Just the thought of getting out of bed, washing and dressing and going into the kitchen for breakfast was daunting. But you summoned up your sinews and drew on your last reserves to make this effort. And now you'll know it was worthwhile.

what you've achieved

▶ You're asleep when your head hits the pillow and awake and out of bed before the alarm rings next morning

▶ You've cleansed your body of the environmental, food and chemical wastes that were slowing down your mental processes, sapping your strength and burning your energy

▶ You've rested your liver and drastically lightened its load so it can start getting rid of the toxic chemicals stored in its fat deposits

▶ You've improved the overall efficiency of your body's chemistry and so kick-started the process whereby energy begets more energy

▶ You've increased your powers of strength, stamina and endurance, and you're now prepared to cope with anything that life throws in your path.

how you feel

I know you'll be feeling extremely proud – proud of your courage to even start on a detox and proud of your perseverance and determination in seeing it through. You're now deservedly rewarded and set to enjoy those rewards for a long time to come:

▶ For the first time that you can remember in ages, you get out of bed feeling full of energy to face the day ahead

▶ You feel sharp and alert, with great mental focus

▶ Your concentration and perception are working well and you're finding it much easier to make decisions and stick to them. When your energy levels were low it was far more difficult to make up your mind and even harder to have faith in the decisions that you eventually came to

▶ On a physical level, you feel more energetic than you have for years. Suddenly you want to get on with all those odd jobs you've been putting off – mending the broken cupboard door, cleaning out the garage, tidying up the garden, or finally clearing all the old clothes out of your wardrobe.

▶ On a social level, you now feel able to renew contact with old friends, make those phone calls, accept invitations and rejoin the land of the energetic living.

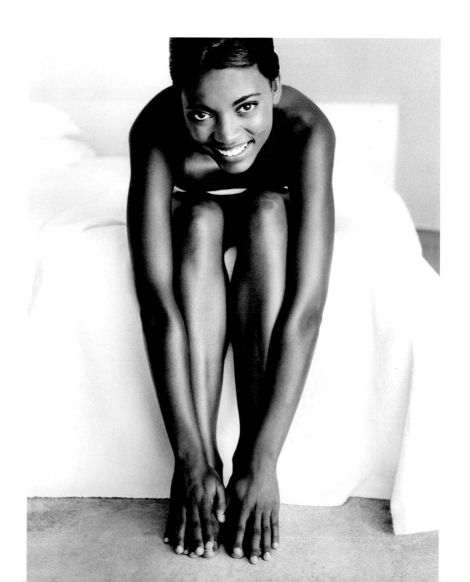

replenishing for

All your efforts in completing the cleansing detox will be wasted if you just return to your old bad habits, so what you need now is to make up your energy deficit and replenish your depleted stores. It's extremely important that you resist the temptation to take the easy way out and stuff yourself on high-energy foods and drinks. All these do is provide large amounts of sugar and little else.

From now on, you need to plan your eating so that your energy supplies always match your energy requirements as closely as possible. That's the way to avoid getting back into your old bad habits. You only need to run out of petrol at three o'clock in the morning once in your life to make sure that you keep your tank well topped up for ever after. And I hope you've now learnt the same lesson regarding your body's fuel tank.

the importance of mental energy

Most people fail to recognise that mental energy and physical energy are equally important. While your physical energy can be replenished through the sugar in your bloodstream, you can also replenish your reserves of mental energy.

The first step is to learn to be more assertive and to actually say 'no' when people ask you to take on extra jobs at home, work or in your leisure life. So at weekends, don't commit yourself to endless DIY jobs, helping your best friend to move house or cutting your mother-in-law's grass. If you've got a garden, sit in it with a long drink and a good book. Go for a picnic or a walk in the countryside, or see a film or a concert. In other words, get yourself some spiritual as well as physical sustenance.

energy

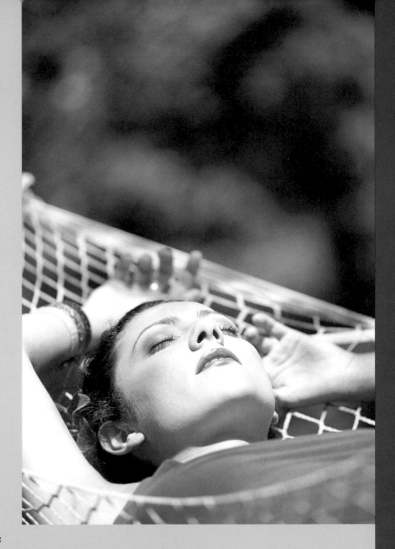

Most of us find it hard to say 'no', but you have to learn to do so. When you do, it may come as a shock to your friends, colleagues and family as they're probably used to you being the one who's always there to help out when there's extra work to do. But try it and you'll be thrilled at how quickly your initial guilt turns to relief and then to self-congratulation.

And as well as giving yourself fewer commitments and so less pressure, what you also need now to help you replenish your energy is regular hours and plenty of good-quality sleep. Once or twice a week have an early supper, a long soak in the bath and be in bed by nine o'clock. Even if you read or listen to the radio in bed, the extra hours of relaxation that you'll enjoy will deliver an energy-boosting charge to your system.

energy through relaxation

Relaxation exercises and meditation are other great ways to replenish your energy. I give some suggested exercises on pages 66–69, but it's worth looking at these now and getting in a little practice as these techniques get much easier with regular use and will help you at this stage of your energizing process as well as later on.

seven-day replenishing

The foods of the next seven days will supply you with both instant- and slow-release energy. This means that your metabolic processes will generate the power necessary for the essential bodily functions, for your immediate physical needs and to build up the surplus that's necessary for your reserve supplies. It's these reserves that help your body cope with sudden emergencies, the unexpected extra demands that crop up every day.

It's important during this week that you eat a little less at a time and do it more often. And to guarantee as wide a spread as possible of energy-giving nutrients, you have to avoid eating the same foods every day. As with the eight-day return to normal eating, if it suits your lifestyle, you can swap a day's meals around, or you can swap whole days, but don't mix meals from different days.

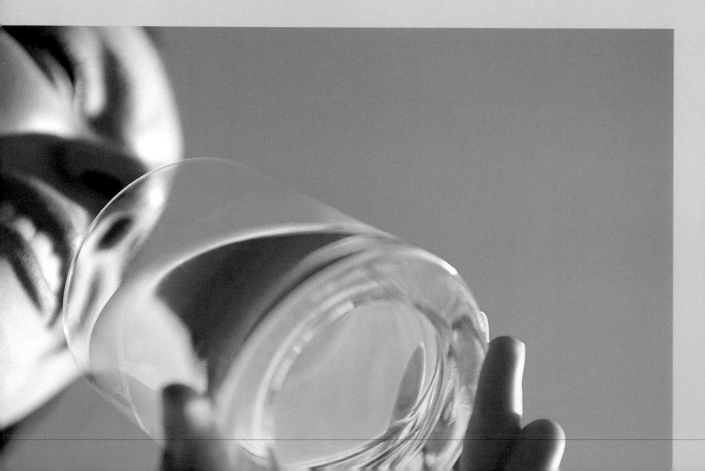

time for a drink

Continue to drink at least 1.5 litres a day, of which at least 1 litre must be water and you can also now drink a total of 5 cups of real tea and coffee, but not more than 3 of coffee. Some alcohol's allowed, but don't exceed 14 units a week if you're a woman, or 21 if you're a man, and carry on avoiding energy-robbing high-sugar canned fizzy drinks.

added extras

Carry on taking your guarana, coenzyme Q, ginseng and vitamin B complex supplements, but now add the following three:

▶ Chromium picolinate helps balance insulin levels
▶ Kelp contains iodine, which you need if your thyroid gland is under-performing
▶ BioStrath Elixir, the universally available Swiss natural herbal tonic

day 1

breakfast Real Swiss Muesli (see recipe, page 80) and a slice of wholemeal toast with honey

mid-morning A selection of dried fruits and fresh unsalted nuts

light meal Wholemeal bread, a selection of cheeses, radishes, celery and fresh fruit

mid-afternoon 1 banana

main meal Large Grilled Prawns on Salad Leaves (see recipe, page 86) with a salad of avocado, spinach and toasted pumpkin seeds
Fresh fruit

day 2

breakfast Dried Fruit Compôte (see recipe, page 105)

mid-morning A matchbox-sized piece of cheese and an apple

light meal Hummous and Guacamole (see recipes, page 102) with hot wholemeal pitta and a selection of crudités

mid-afternoon A mixture of raisins and unsalted, unroasted peanuts

main meal Spicy Energy Beans (see recipe, page 91)
Tomato and Red Onion Salad (see recipe, page 101)

day 3

breakfast Carrot, Apple and Celery Juice (see recipe, page 85), 2 boiled eggs and 2 slices of
wholemeal toast with butter

mid-morning Yoghurt and Fruit Smoothie (see recipe, page 85)

light meal Leek and Potato Soup (see recipe, page 99) with wholemeal bread and a bunch of grapes

mid-afternoon Pitta bread and Hummous (see recipe, page 102)

main meal Steak in Red Wine (see recipe, page 91)

day 4

breakfast Buckwheat Crêpes (see recipe, page 82)

mid-morning Rye crispbread with cottage cheese and a few dates

light meal Mediterranean Omelette Flan (see recipe, page 86)

mid-afternoon Greek yoghurt with a teaspoon of honey and sunflower seeds

main meal Millet and Mushroom Risotto (see recipe, page 89)
Spiced Baked Apple (see recipe, page 104)

day 5

breakfast Scrambled Eggs with Smoked Salmon (see recipe, page 81) on wholemeal toast
A glass of half-orange and half-grapefruit juice

mid-morning	Dried fruit with fresh unsalted nuts
light meal	Gratin of Potatoes and Mushrooms (see recipe, page 89)
mid-afternoon	Energy Teabread (see recipe, page 80)
main meal	Dutch Chicken (see recipe, page 87) with rice Honeyed Plums (see recipe, page 105) with crème fraîche

day 6

breakfast	A glass of tomato juice, fresh fruit salad – use any seasonal fruits – a carton of live yoghurt and 1 slice of wholemeal toast
mid-morning	Apple, Peanut and Banana Smoothie (see recipe, page 85)
light meal	Tuna and Mixed Bean Salad (see recipe, page 101)
mid-afternoon	Dried Fruit Compôte (see recipe, page 105)
main meal	Baked Cod with Sesame Seeds (see recipe, page 91) Mango and Kiwi Sorbet (see recipe, page 104)

day 7

breakfast	Savoury Toastie (see recipe, page 82)
mid-morning	Energy Teabread (see recipe, page 80)
light meal	Chillied Sardine Sandwiches (see recipe, page 89) with cherry tomatoes and watercress
mid-afternoon	Small bowl of Real Swiss Muesli (see recipe, page 80)
main meal	Beef Stir-Fry (see recipe, page 92) served on a bed of noodles Banana and Mango Crumble (see recipe, page 105)

replenishing summary

Now things are really starting to hum. Your overall food consumption is better balanced than ever before and as a result you feel you can take on the world, whether at home, at work or in your social life. Everyone around you can detect that buzz of energy and aura of vitality. In fact, they're all having trouble keeping up with you.

what you've achieved

Thanks to the replenishing programme, your life is now on a more even keel and you've managed to smooth out the peaks and troughs that have been such a feature of your blood-sugar patterns for longer than you care to remember.

It's natural that you may not have liked all the dishes I've suggested, but by now you should understand the nutritional principles behind the Super Energy Detox. You may even have made appropriate substitutions with foods that you enjoy. If you've done it correctly:

▶ Your energy levels will have increased enough to make you more energetic both physically and mentally
▶ You will have removed most of the stress to your body's insulin/sugar mechanisms, which in turn can help reduce your risk of developing Type II diabetes (Non-Insulin Dependent Diabetes) in later life
▶ You should be performing better at work thanks to improved concentration and more efficient short-term memory
▶ You have arrived at a major turning point in the status of your general health. By making up for years of energy deficit and by replenishing your energy stores, you've set the scene for rebuilding your energy. This is the last step before you start to plan the rest of your life for energy.

how you feel

You've done exceptionally well to get this far and the rewards are obvious to you and to everyone else:

▶ You feel great about yourself and can't wait to get on with things. In fact, you may even find yourself getting a bit impatient with others around you who are less energetic

▶ Although you feel the buzz of replenished energy, you're not agitated or hyperactive. On the contrary, you feel an inner calm because you know you can cope with any mental or physical demands

▶ Because you no longer suffer the violent mood swings that were related to your chronic fatigue, you feel happier and much less worried about your temper. You've stopped flying off the handle for no real reason, which makes relationships with your nearest and dearest easier and much more pleasant

▶ Surprisingly, you're feeling much better behind the wheel of your car. Although you may still believe that everyone else on the road is an idiot, you've stopped waving your fists, you let other cars into the traffic flow and you haven't used the horn for ages.

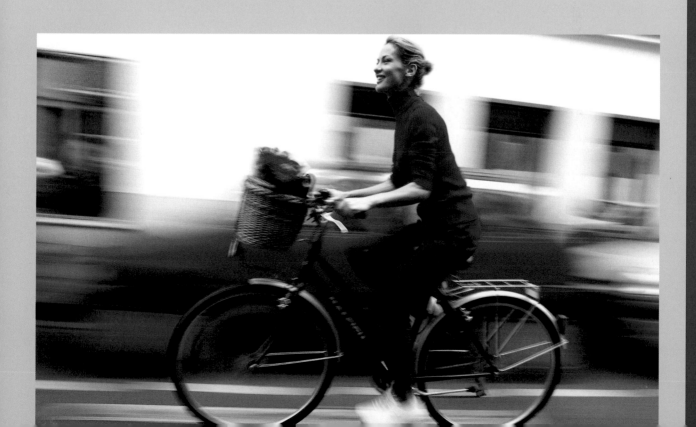

rebuilding for

At last, the moment you've been waiting for – when you start to rebuild your energy and generate a pattern that will sustain you in the future. These next steps will lay the foundations for Part 2's Super Energy for Life.

the bad guys/good guys swap box

One thing you can do to help you improve your energy levels is to make some simple changes to your normal eating habits. When it comes to food, there are good guys and bad guys. Choosing to eat the good guys will start you on the road to rebuilding your energy faster than you think, but there is an important added bonus. By reducing the amount of high-fat, high-salt, high-sugar foods that you consume on a regular basis and by increasing your consumption of whole grains, nuts, seeds and complex carbohydrates, you reduce your risk of heart disease, circulatory disorders and many types of cancer.

BAD GUYS	GOOD GUYS
Sugar-coated cereals	Porridge, muesli, wholewheat cereal
Meat pies, pasties, salamis	Fish, organic beef, lamb, poultry
Biscuits, sweets, chocolates	Dried fruit, bananas
Chips	Baked or boiled potatoes
Salty snacks	Fresh nuts and seeds
Sliced white bread	Organic wholemeal or rye
Convenience foods	Simple home cooking
Burgers and hot dogs	Veggie pizza, shish kebab in pitta
Squashes, fizzy drinks	Water, fresh juices

See, it's not as hard as you thought.

energy

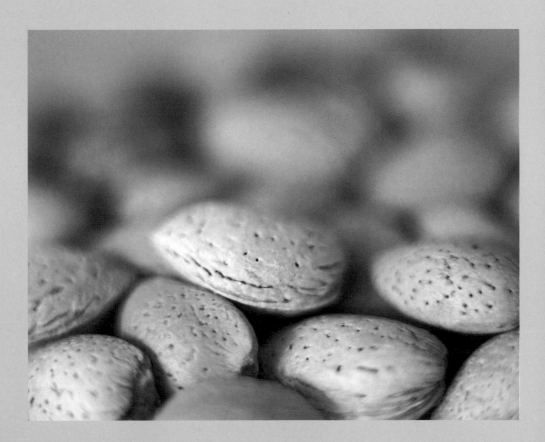

the zinc problem

Chronic fatigue has become an epidemic. If you've suffered exhaustion for several weeks, you must see your doctor in case an underlying medical condition like anaemia, a thyroid problem or diabetes is responsible. Zinc deficiency is a common cause of exhaustion, but excessive tiredness is also a symptom of depression, so many doctors are likely to prescribe anti-depressants. But anti-depressants interfere with the body's absorption of zinc, so you end up in a vicious circle. Forewarned is forearmed.

fourteen-day rebuilding

Start this Rebuilding for Energy regime with the seven-day Replenishing for Energy eating plan. It will help get you into the right frame of mind as well as into the routine of eating properly for energy. In other words, it will introduce you to the concept of grazing, which helps you maintain a constant blood-sugar level and so avoid the ups and downs that drain your energy resources so severely.

Throughout this second week you may choose any of the mid-morning or mid-afternoon snacks from the first week – but please don't just rely on your favourite two or three. Ringing the changes spreads your nutritional input so you obtain the optimum amounts of essential vitamins, minerals and protective plant chemicals.

drinks

▶ As with the Replenishing for Energy programme, still maintain a high level of fluid intake – at least one and a half litres a day, one litre of which should be water.

▶ Indian tea and real coffee are allowed, but not more than 5 cups day and certainly not more than 3 cups of coffee – avoiding instant decaffeinated coffee of course.

▶ Some alcohol is still allowed, but not more than 4 units a week for a woman, 21 for a man.

▶ Don't drink canned fizzy drinks of any kind. They're either full of energy-robbing sugar or full of chemical artificial sweeteners. Yuk!

Days 1–7, follow the Seven-Day Replenishing programme.

day 8

breakfast Porridge with Cinnamon and Dried Fruits (see recipe, page 80)
1 slice of wholemeal toast with a scraping of butter
1 banana
A glass of orange juice

light meal Avocado, Tomato and Mozzarella Salad (see recipe, page 103)

main meal Traditional Chicken Soup (see recipe, page 100)
Squash, Almond and Raisin Bulgur (see recipe, page 93)
Dried Fruit Compôte (see recipe, page 105)

day 9

breakfast Lightly cooked fresh fruit compôte of strawberries, raspberries, currants, blackberries, blueberries and apple with plain live yoghurt
1 boiled egg
1 slice of wholemeal toast with butter

light meal Channel Island Potato Salad (see recipe, page 103)
A piece of fresh fruit

main meal Posh Cauliflower Cheese with Pasta (see recipe, page 94)
Tomato and Red Onion Salad (see recipe, page 101)
Orange and Mango Fool (see recipe, page 104)

day 10

breakfast 1 whole pink grapefruit
3–4 canned (in olive oil) sardines mashed with black pepper and lemon juice, spread on 2 slices of wholemeal toast and covered with sliced tomato

light meal Pasta all'Aglio e Olio (see recipe, page 87) with mixed green salad

main meal   1 slice of fresh ogen or cantaloupe melon
Roman Liver (see recipe, page 95) with runner beans and carrots
Oatcakes, goat's cheese and a bunch of grapes

day 11
breakfast   A glass of half-orange, half-grapefruit juice
Real Swiss Muesli (see recipe, page 80) sprinkled with 1 teaspoon each of sunflower,
sesame and pumpkin seeds

light meal   Wholemeal pitta stuffed with tomato, cucumber, radishes, spring onion, shredded lettuce,
celery, watercress and olives, with a drizzle of good extra-virgin olive oil and a sprinkling
of oregano
A piece of fresh fruit

main meal   A glass of tomato juice
Baked Cod with Sesame Seeds (see recipe, page 91) on a bed of spinach
Bread and Tomato Salad (see recipe, page 100)
A bowl of fresh strawberries

day 12
breakfast   A glass of beetroot juice
Mushrooms on Wholemeal Toast (see recipe, page 81)

light meal   A large jacket potato filled with baked beans
A glass of pineapple juice
Fresh cherries and a bunch of grapes

main meal   Grilled Lamb Cutlets with Rosemary (see recipe, page 94) with boiled new potatoes in
their skins and kale
Dried Fruit Compôte (see recipe, page 105) with Greek yoghurt

day 13

breakfast Fresh orange, pink grapefruit, tangerine and kiwi slices with natural live yoghurt sprinkled with a tablespoon of flaked almonds and a drizzle of honey
Poached Kipper and Tomato (see recipe, page 83)
1 slice of wholemeal toast

light meal Lamb and Pine-Kernel Koftas (see recipe, page 92) with a salad of watercress, mint and chopped onion

main meal Brown Rice Risotto with Sun-dried Tomatoes (see recipe, page 94) served with Spanish Salad (see recipe, page 101)
Spiced Baked Apple (see recipe, page 104)

day 14

breakfast English Breakfast the Healthy Way (see recipe, page 83)

light meal Ten-Minute Mussels (see recipe, page 93) with crusty French bread
1 pear

main meal Duck Breasts with Pepper Sauce (see recipe, page 95) served with Grilled Italian Vegetables (see recipe, page 95)
1 peach

rebuilding summary

If you've got this far, you'll have achieved the remarkable feat of turning your life around and preparing yourself to enjoy the rest of it with boundless super energy. Chinese takeaways, burgers and chips, buckets of fried chicken and high-fat, high-gristle and high-salt meat pies are all things of the past.

By now you've almost certainly completely changed your eating habits and I hope that the diet plans so far have got you in the kitchen and started you cooking. Hopefully, you'll also have discovered the pleasure of shopping for food and preparing it at home from fresh natural ingredients.

what you've achieved

▶ You have become much more knowledgeable about food and with a bit of luck, you'll have made friends with the butcher, the baker, the fishmonger and the greengrocer. Even if you only shop for food in supermarkets, you'll find that they have experts you can talk to who are always happy to give advice, discuss recipes and tell you the best way to cook what they have available

▶ You have become much more discerning and critical when you shop. When you do the cooking you soon spot the tired vegetables, the not-so-fresh fish, the fatty cut of meat and the fruit which has been in cold store so long that it rots before it ripens

▶ You have developed a whole range of cooking skills you never had before. The terms sauté, sweat, steam and stir-fry trip off your tongue as if you were a celebrity Michelin-starred chef

▶ You have learnt enough about your energy needs to be able to plan a day's menus without needing the guidance in this book. You are already thinking ahead so you can cook today food that will last for tomorrow and the next day. Your store cupboard never runs out of the basic essentials, so you can always throw together delicious, nourishing and energising meals with whatever comes to hand.

how you feel

▶ Vibrant and energetic describes what you're feeling now. You're probably thinking of running the next marathon for your favourite charity – but please don't! As an osteopath I can tell you that marathon running is a health disaster and guaranteed to damage your ankles, knees, hips and spine

▶ You feel surprised at the enormous change in your outlook and energy. Even though you'll get used to this feeling, try not to take it for granted. Just remember how you once were and don't stop taking care of your energy levels

▶ You feel very smug, and you're certainly entitled to. Every time you watch others pushing their trolleys full of convenience foods, frozen burgers, cases of fizzy drinks and sliced wrapped bread through the checkout, you find it hard to believe that you ever did the same.

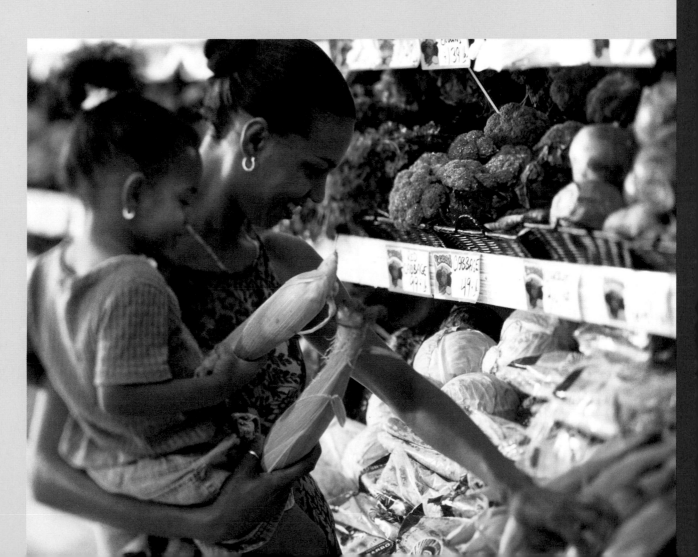

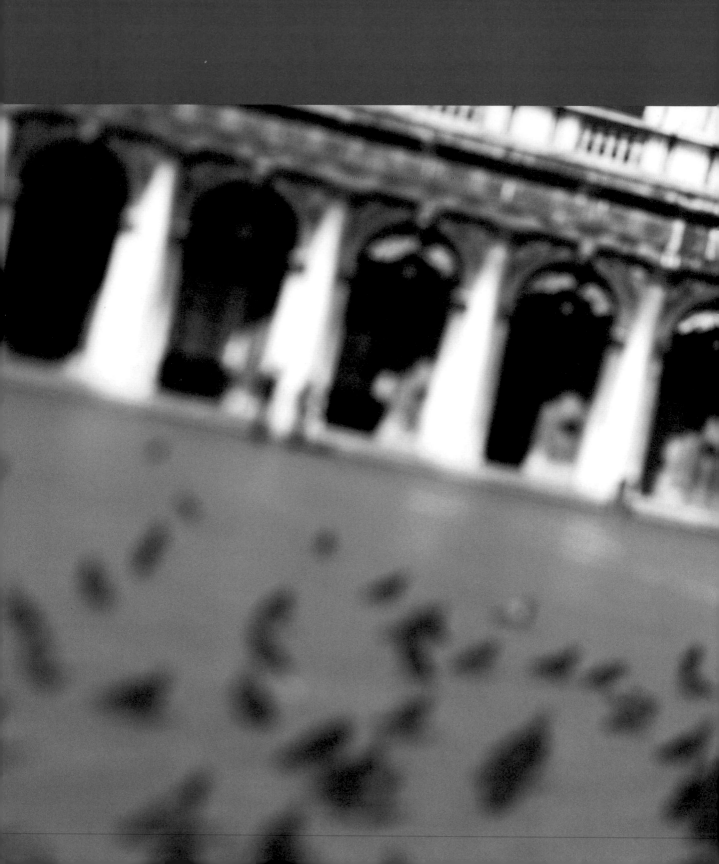

part 2 super energy for life

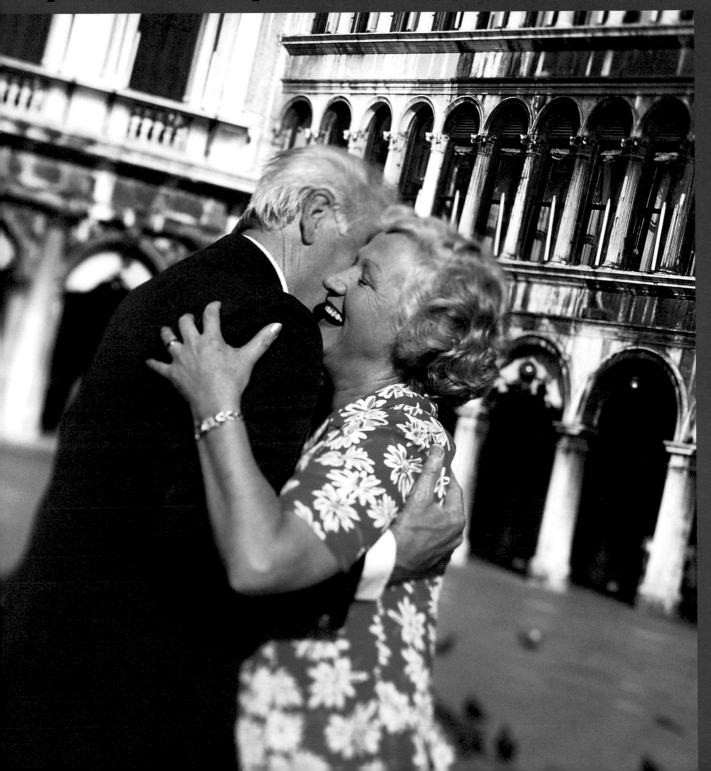

energy lifeplan

It's inevitable to experience an occasional attack of the energy-droops – too many late nights, a few drinks too many, a time of extra pressure at work, problems at home, or even the after-effects of a cold or of an attack of flu. If you're healthy you'll soon recover from these episodes, or you could give yourself a detox to help you get back on your feet.

But to avoid regular and frequent troughs, you need to plan your life for energy. It doesn't matter whether it's the energy you need for your day-to-day activities at home, for that immediate burst of extra zap required for a particularly hard day at work, or enough energy to extract maximum pleasure and enjoyment from your leisure activities.

Whatever your requirements, this chapter will tell you how to keep your body's supplies of essential vitality at a constant level. No more peaks and troughs. No more periods of being mentally hyper – the only way you've been able to cope in the past but it drives everyone around you crazy. No more superhuman efforts to drag yourself up from the depths of total exhaustion and conceal your chronic fatigue by putting on a brave face.

The lifestyle changes for energy at home, work and leisure that I suggest will help you generate all the energy you need and will ensure that you've always got a bit in reserve for emergencies.

ten-point plan for lifestyle changes at home for energy

To achieve your goal of a high-energy home life you may need to follow all ten of these steps or you may need just a few of them. They're simple and effective and won't make too many demands on your already low energy levels.

1 Clear the clutter – there is nothing so fatiguing as living in a constant muddle. Fight against the magpie instinct and stop being a hoarder. Get rid of stuff you don't need.

2 Make sure your home is well ventilated and turn the heating down a couple of degrees. More fresh air and a cooler temperature help generate more physical energy.

3 Think about redecorating. Drab colours make for drab people – beige is enervating. You don't have to use crimson and gold, but lively colours generate their own energy.

4 Check all heating appliances annually as low levels of carbon monoxide from unserviced heaters are a common cause of chronic fatigue and high levels could be fatal.

5 Fresh flowers in the house are great givers of energy – a vase of daffodils in the spring, wild hedgerow flowers in the summer, a few twigs of autumn leaves or a bowl of scented hyacinths at Christmas are all signs of Nature's vigour.

6 Turn your bathroom into a spa by adding invigorating essential oils like rosemary, pine or eucalyptus to your bath.

7 Cold baths or showers are very stimulating and push the body into producing extra energy. When you've finished washing, slowly add cold water to the bath while rubbing your arms, legs and stomach briskly with a rough flannel or loofah. If you're having a shower, turn the temperature down gradually. Once the water is really cold, stay in it for at least 10 seconds then dry yourself as briskly as possible with a rough towel. You may think it sounds awful, but once you've tried it you'll be hooked.

8 Fragrance your home with genuine herbal pot pourri and banish forever artificially scented air fresheners, fake aromatherapy candles and room deodorisers – the synthetic musk perfumes they contain are all toxic and de-energizing.

9 A good night's sleep is vital for energy at home, so make sure your bedroom has curtains which exclude all light and if necessary put lightproof roller blinds behind them.

10 Check your mattress. In 20 years you may have bought 5 toasters, 3 irons and 6 cars, and still be sleeping on the same mattress. Once it sags, it won't support you properly and you won't get the restful, energy-generating sleep you need.

the power of breakfast

While you sleep your body is working hard as this is the time for growth and repair. Your brain switches off the activity hormones and turns on to maintenance mode. While all this work is going on you are using up your reserves of vital nutrients, so your storehouse needs replenishing, which is why breakfast is the most important meal of the day.

The ancient proverb 'Breakfast like a king, lunch like a prince, dine like a pauper' has more than a grain of truth in it, but sadly most people today skip breakfast altogether. This is really bad news as ideally you should be getting 25 per cent of your day's calories from breakfast. It is exactly what it says, breaking your fast, and for most people the time they spend in bed is the longest period they go without food. When you get up in the morning it may be 8–12 hours since you last ate and your blood-sugar level is at rock bottom. In order for your brain to function properly it needs a constant supply of sugar, which is why starting your day with breakfast is so important.

Skipping breakfast means poorer performance by schoolchildren, a greater risk of accidents when driving, and a lack of efficiency at work. It also means irritability.

scary statistics

Five million people don't bother to eat breakfast but grab a snack while dashing to work. Then they consume one and a half million bacon sandwiches, over a million packets of crisps, more than a million sugary soft drinks and half a million bags of sweets or bars of chocolate. Worse still, half of people at work don't eat anything for breakfast at all.

breakfast rules

What you eat for breakfast depends on your needs for that particular morning. Replenishing your protein means real energy and brain activity, whereas a mainly starch-based breakfast keeps you calm, serene and happy.

the sporting breakfast

If you take your exercise early in the day, the essential ingredient in your breakfast should be lots of healthy calories and a fairly modest amount of protein, so the ideal start for you is a large bowl of porridge or muesli with 3 prunes, 3 dried apricots, a handful of sultanas or raisins and a generous sprinkling of mixed sunflower and pumpkin seeds for extra minerals. Follow with a matchbox-sized piece of cheese and an apple, and take a banana with you to replace the energy and potassium after your exercise.

the expectant breakfast

Pregnancy isn't the time to think about dieting. As well as extra energy you need extra nutrients. A small pot of plain live yoghurt with a generous dessertspoon of runny honey drizzled on the top and a sprinkling of mixed chopped, unsalted, unroasted fresh nuts will get you off to a good start in the morning. This will provide energy, protein, calcium, vitamin E and lots of other essential nutrients. Follow with at least 1 thick slice of good wholemeal or rye toast spread with organic peanut butter – yes, it's extremely healthy and a great source of instant energy – and a glass of fresh unsweetened fruit juice or unsalted vegetable juice.

the business power breakfast

If you're straight into a high-powered meeting that requires your brain to be bursting with energy, you need a high-protein breakfast, but avoid the traditional high-fat, high-cholesterol, artery-clogging frying pan breakfast, and skip the waffles and cream. Poached eggs, griddled bacon, a grilled low-fat sausage with grilled tomatoes and mushrooms, a glass of juice, and 2 slices of good wholemeal toast will get you off to a flying start. The protein will stimulate your brain activity and energetic thought and you'll be unstoppable!

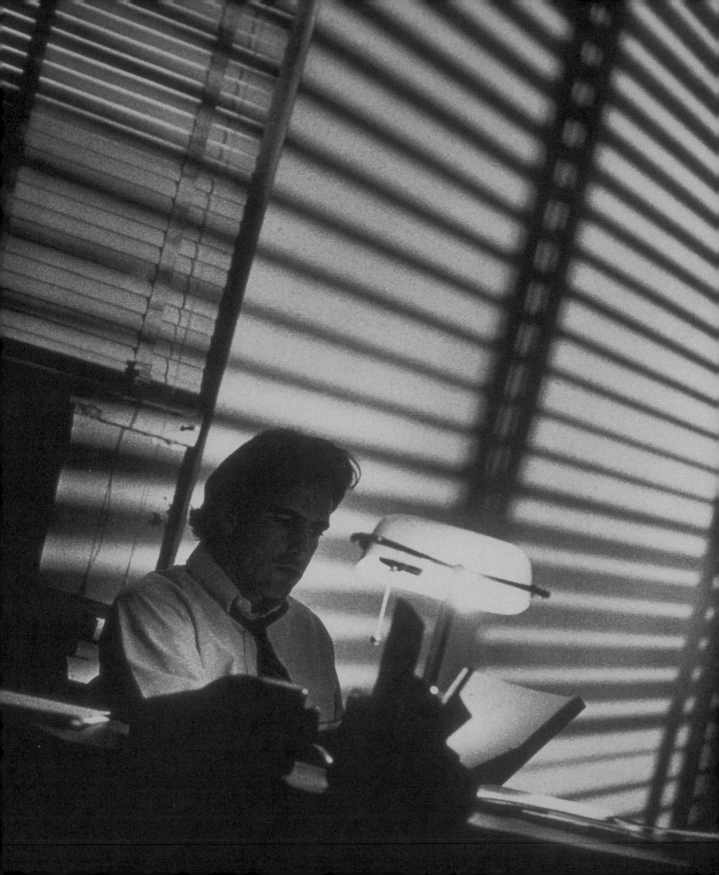

lifestyle changes at work

Everyone needs energy to do their job and depending on what you do, it may be physical energy, mental energy or, in most situations, a combination of the two. It's impossible to perform at your optimum level if you're constantly tired, but this is all too common a situation for many people in the workplace.

Assuming there's no underlying medical cause for your lack of energy, it's nearly always the result of a poor working environment, bad working posture, ergonomically wrong workstations and equipment or, all too commonly, just plain boredom. If you dislike your job, it's hard to summon up any enthusiasm. If you have to put up with bullying or sexual harassment from colleagues or superiors, you will inevitably be depressed, and fatigue goes hand in hand with depression.

I've already explained the vital role that nutrition plays in the production of usable energy, and at work nutrition is even more important. You must not let the pressures of the job prevent you eating at regular intervals and you won't manage to break through the fatigue barrier if you're constantly relying on high-sugar snacks to give you an artificial energy boost.

Everyone wants to enjoy the satisfaction of a job well done and to achieve it you need to work in the most efficient way. To do that you must have energy in abundance and this will only be generated when you're reasonably happy and able to work in comfort.

ten-point plan for lifestyle changes at work for energy

Here's your ten-point plan for lifestyle changes that will maximize your energy at work.

1 All high-energy work days must start with a good breakfast.

2 With air conditioning in the summer and central heating in the winter, most work places are drier than the Sahara desert. This causes you to dehydrate and nothing saps your energy as quickly. Make sure you drink at least one and a half litres of water between arriving at work and going home. You'll feel more comfortable generally and will be less at risk of getting headaches, which are exhausting in themselves.

3 Electronic machinery such as computers and printers pump out ozone and tiny particulates of carbon which irritate the eyes, lungs and other mucus membranes. Create your own micro-climate by surrounding your workspace with loads of green plants, particularly ivies and spider plants. Plants not only give off moisture, which increases humidity and makes the atmosphere more comfortable, but they absorb pollutants too.

4 Always switch off electrical appliances when they're not being used. If you leave them in standby mode, they still produce ozone. The increase in your energy levels will more than compensate for the moments you have to wait for them to warm up.

5 If you use a computer for long periods you need a kitchen timer. Set it for 30 minutes and when it pings, sit back in your chair, look out of the window or across the room, and give your eyes and brain a 2-minute break. In addition, make sure you look away from the screen for at least 30 seconds every 15 minutes and focus your eyes on a distant object.

6 If your job frequently requires you to use a keyboard and the telephone at the same time, you must insist on having a hands- free headset. Keeping the telephone wedged between your ear and your shoulder while you access or input data is an almost certain guarantee of headaches, stiff necks, painful shoulders, backache and constant fatigue.

7 You must take the time to organise your desk or workstation to suit you – it's no good having the telephone on the right-hand side if you're left-handed. Make sure you have an ergonomic chair that is fully adjustable to suit your size and shape, and that you have a footstool. This will maximise your comfort, minimise muscular effort and conserve your much-needed energy.

8 Take the opportunity of your lunch break to recharge your energy reserves. Don't sit at your desk with a sandwich but get out of the office, even if it is raining. A short walk stimulates your circulation and breathing, which increases oxygen levels and stimulates your metabolism to produce more energy.

9 As well as eating all the energy superfoods (see pages 8–9), you must also eat to beat office pollution. That's not just chemicals and irritants, but also the myriad viruses and bacteria that circulate through the heating and cooling systems. To boost your natural resistance and protect you against infections which will drastically reduce your energy levels, eat a generous portion of at least two of these foods every day: carrots, red or yellow peppers, apricots, strawberries, blackberries, blueberries, spinach, watercress, spring greens, broccoli, sweet potatoes, cantaloupe melon, tomatoes, and dark green or red lettuce.

10 When you sit for long periods, your entire circulatory system slows down. This reduces the supply of oxygen to the brain and is a major contributor to office fatigue. Get into the habit of standing up during telephone calls. Shift your weight from foot to foot, do some gentle knee bends, take a few steps each way, stand on tiptoe a few times – all of this works the muscle pump in your calves and stimulates better blood flow.

last but not least

It's all too easy to forget that mental energy is as important as physical energy at work. Just as a 10-minute catnap can restore your physical activity levels, so a few minutes spent in simple meditation can stimulate an immediate increase in your mental energy. Surprisingly, this type of mental and spiritual relaxation doesn't leave you feeling down and sleepy, but can help set you up for the rest of the day's work (see pages 68–69).

lifestyle changes at leisure

We often equate leisure with relaxation and unwinding, which is quite proper as it should be both. But it is important to understand that by using your leisure time constructively, you can really recharge your body's batteries. This process not only generates the immediate energy you need to enjoy your leisure pursuits, but also fills your energy tank to overflowing, allowing the surplus to be carried over into your home and working life.

I discuss in detail the vital relationship between leisure, pleasure and health in this book's companion volume, Super Health Detox. But without a shadow of doubt, if you want to stimulate and release both your mental and physical energy, the key is how you spend your leisure time.

Ideally you should cultivate a combination of intellectual and physical leisure activities. This gives you a holistic energy boost that activates mind and body. After all, it's not much use if the spirit is willing but the flesh is weak, or conversely, if you're bursting with physical energy and so mentally exhausted that you can't even take the first step.

Chairman Mao was fond of saying that a march of a thousand kilometres begins with a single step. Bear this in mind and use it as the spur you need to take that first step into a new world of energy-boosting leisure activities. Don't worry about how you'll cope after 10 kilometres. Just focus on putting one foot in front of the other. You'll be surprised at how quickly you become absorbed in what you're doing, and that will be the beginning of the regeneration of your energy.

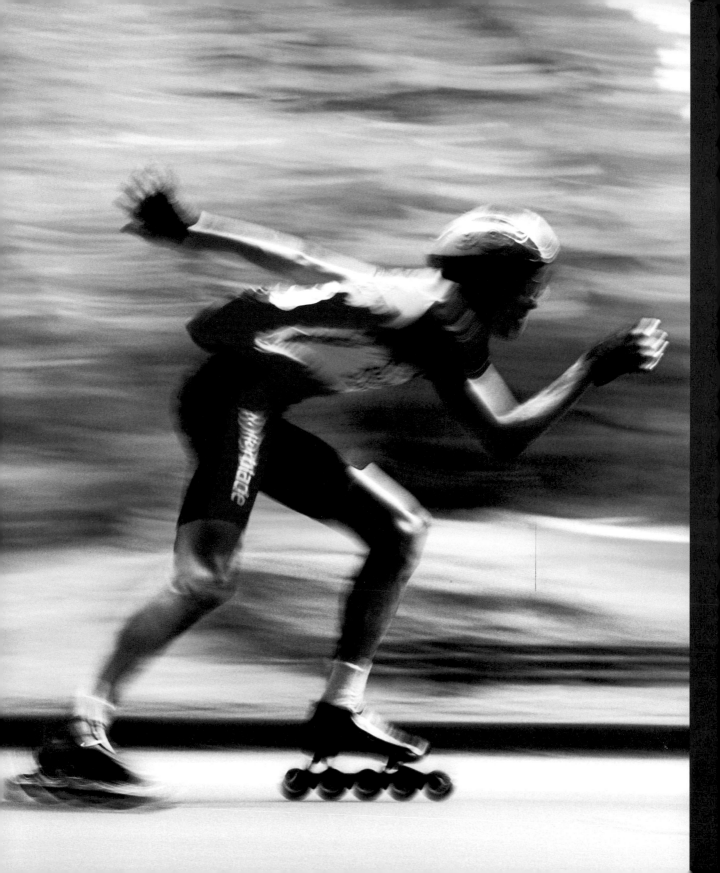

ten-point plan for lifestyle changes at leisure for energy

If you don't have any leisure time, it's your own fault and if you have it but don't use it properly, that's your own fault too. Don't forget that all work and no play makes Jack a dull and tired boy and in today's world, it's likely to be just as true, if not more true, for Jill as well. Feeling energetic is one of the really good things in life and the good things are worth struggling for.

This ten-point action plan will make the struggle a great deal easier and the prize at the end is worth more than a pot of gold. You'll have a boundless supply of energy which will let you enjoy your leisure to the full.

1 Prioritize your time. Work out a schedule and allocate at least five hours in each working week as private leisure time – and that doesn't include your lunch hour or the time you spend travelling to and from work.

2 At weekends you must set aside at least one continuous three-hour period or two sets of two hours for leisure activities on your own or with friends and family.

3 Use some of your leisure time for relaxation exercises. These will give your mental and emotional energy an immediate boost (see page 66). Contrary to popular belief, mental therapies like yoga, meditation, visualization, self-hypnosis and even prayer, are all great stress-busters, which is why they are so effective. Emotional tension creates anxiety, which triggers excessive production of the hormone adrenaline. This prepares the body for fight or flight, which in turn causes muscle tension. Prolonged periods of this type of stress mean that your muscles are constantly ready for action and permanently in a state of contraction, and this results in pain, discomfort and the relentless burning up of your energy reserves by all that muscular effort.

4 Make sure you channel some of your leisure time into cultural activities as these are another key to good mental energy. It makes no difference at all whether your cultural activities consist of going to pop festivals, discos and clubs, or visiting art galleries, listening to chamber music or going to the opera. It doesn't matter whether you prefer to read sex-and-shopping novels, sci-fi and mysteries, or philosophy, the classics and historical novels. What is important is satisfying your spiritual need for cultural stimulus.

5 Another great source of mental energy is playing games. This is also a brilliant way of building relationships with friends, family and children. You must choose a game that's appropriate to your playing companions, but it absolutely doesn't matter whether it's snap or bridge, Monopoly or Scrabble, snakes and ladders or tiddlywinks, charades or Trivial Pursuits. Any of these games will shake up the grey matter and, win or lose, will give you a mental-energy boost. Just keep away from the computer and the Game Boy.

6 Now it's time to get physical. I always have problems when I tell patients who suffer from chronic fatigue that they need to take some physical exercise, as it's the last thing they feel like doing. But getting the body moving releases the feelgood hormones in the brain and the energy-packing activity hormones in the rest of the body. No matter how tired you feel when you get home from work, do something physical.

7 Choose appropriate exercise. If you're looking for a burst of super energy on a regular basis, you have to choose a form of activity that is appropriate to your age and general health. If you've been a couch potato for years, don't start with advanced aerobics or long-distance running. Begin slowly and build up to three regular sessions of 20–30 minutes a week. Even a brisk walk – enough to make you sweat and get home slightly out of breath – will start the process off.

8 Choose exercise you enjoy – if you hate it you'll never keep it up. Ideally, try to ensure you do a different type of exercise for each period of leisure time that you set aside. Walking, swimming and golf would be a great combination. But you can just as well choose tennis, squash, tenpin-bowling, line dancing, folk dancing, cycling, jogging or even gardening. Just remember that the object is to generate energy, and this will happen automatically the more you exercise.

9 If you're getting physical, do take sensible precautions. If you decide to use a mini-scooter, roller blades or a bicycle, then make sure you wear the proper protective gear, as you won't generate much energy lying in a hospital bed with a fractured skull or kneecap.

10 Keep at it. Be committed, be regular and don't allow outside pressures like work to interfere with your leisure time.

the perils of life in the 24/7 society

Isn't it great? You can shop in the supermarket at two in the morning, go on-line, check your bank balance and pay your bills at three, nip round to the all-night garage, fill your tank, have a coffee and a doughnut at four and still get home to watch a movie on satellite TV before it's time to pour the milk on your breakfast cereal. An hour's catnap and you're off to work.

Even the Sunday morning lie-in, followed by a leisurely breakfast with the kids and a family lunch, have vanished. 78 per cent of you are up and doing by nine o'clock, checking your emails, reading your text messages or answering your mobile phone. Then 50 per cent of you go shopping and 25 per cent go to work – what sort of rest is this?

It's not so long ago that in many countries all shops shut for lunch, had one day a week when they closed in the afternoon, and none stayed open all day on Saturday, let alone open at all on Sunday. Sunday really was a day of rest, when everyone could recharge their batteries. But not any more.

shift workers

Because we inhabit the non-stop world of 24/7 living, far more people now have to work shifts and they're the ones that suffer the worst health problems. Professor Neil Stanley, Chairman of the British Sleep Society, is one of the world's experts on conditions caused by disrupted sleep patterns. 'My major concern is accidents,' says the professor. 'World catastrophes like the Exxon Valdez oil spill, the Chernobyl and Three Mile Island nuclear accidents, and the Bhopal chemical explosion in India, all happened in the small hours of the night shift, when people's concentration, alertness and energy were at their lowest ebb.

'It's well documented that driving home after the night shift makes you more likely to have an accident than if you're four times over the alcohol limit, and you're 40 per cent more likely to have any sort of accident, whether it's in the car or at home. There is no doubt that shift work kills you early as well as making you tired.'

the effects on women

Everyone suffers the effects of 24/7 living, but women seem to come off worst. Constant disruptions of regular sleep patterns increase the risk of breast cancer and women working a night shift at least once a week for three years or more have a 60 per cent increased risk. Being exposed to bright light all through the working night increases oestrogen levels, which also upsets the menstrual cycle. This can be the trigger of PMS, irregular periods, fertility problems and, when women do manage to conceive they're more likely to have difficult pregnancies.

the effects on men

The 24/7 lifestyle affects men too and though they may not be in the supermarket in the middle of the night – unless they're working there – they're much more likely to be putting in longer hours at work, sitting up for much of the night surfing the net, or watching sport and adult movies on television.

And according to the British Trades Union Council, when men have to work late into the night, their jobs may put them at greater risk of physical violence. Late-night petrol-pump attendants and small shop, restaurant or takeaway owners and staff are vulnerable when bars and clubs close.

If the men are actually on shift work, their chances of developing serious heart disease go up by a frightening 40 per cent and they're far more likely than other male workers to suffer from lack of energy and chronic fatigue. And on top of that, shift workers commonly have constipation and stomach problems due to dehydration, irregular meals and bad eating habits.

the effects on children

Youngsters aren't immune either. Do you know what your children do once you've gone to bed? Many are on their computers or text-messaging their friends. Play Stations and video and DVD players are in overdrive. No wonder you have a job waking your children in the morning and they haven't got the energy to last the day – they've probably only had three or four hours' sleep. They become disruptive at school, neglect their homework and even fall asleep during lessons. Once their regular sleep patterns are disrupted, it's very hard to re-establish them. Then they suffer energy loss and illness just the same as adults.

circadian rhythms

The human body is programmed to work in sync with day and night, and this circadian rhythm controls all our bodily functions. No matter how long you maintain an irregular lifestyle, with too little sleep and too many waking hours during darkness, you will never cope with it. You can no more adapt your body clock to being awake at night and asleep in daylight than you can make your body adapt to living underwater.

So what are the results of this struggle with nature? Emotional disturbances are common. Irritability, bad moods, over-reacting, flying off the handle, poor memory and concentration are just the beginning. You make silly mistakes when trying to do simple tasks and you may even forget important things like collecting the children from school. Constant exhaustion, chronic fatigue and tired-all-the-time syndrome soon follow and go hand-in-hand with diminishing libido and sex drive. All this can destroy relationships.

Your physical health suffers too. Few people realise that in the middle of the night, when you should be safely tucked up in bed and sleeping, the body's white-cell count drops so your immune defences are less effective. If you've really embraced the 24/7 society, those middle-of-the-night trips to the supermarket mean you are much more vulnerable to the bacteria and viruses you come into contact with there. So it's not surprising that night birds get more coughs, colds and flu.

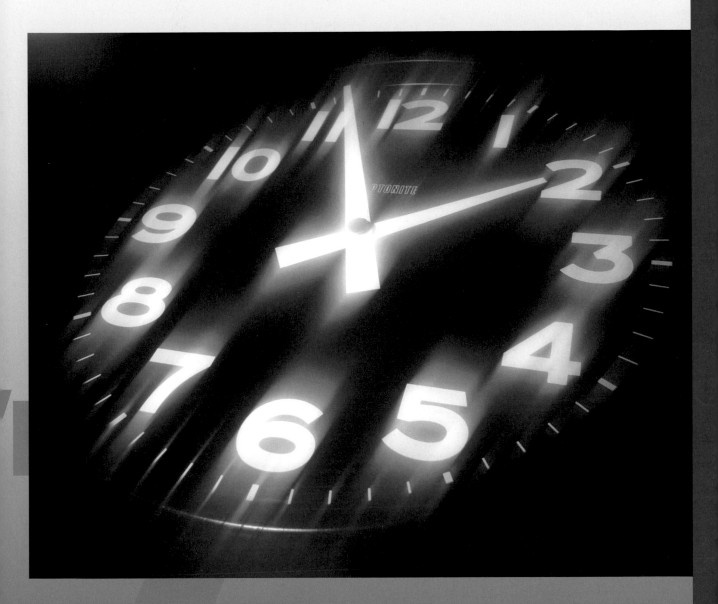

eating to survive the 24/7 world

Living life on the 24/7 treadmill is similar to being jetlagged, but it's results are permanent and they're not going to go away after a few nights' sleep. As your symptoms get worse, you look for crutches and these usually take the form of caffeine and more caffeine, alcohol and more alcohol, cigarettes and more cigarettes. And often, when you finally do decide to go to bed for a few hours, you'll knock back a sleeping pill or two to help you get off to sleep.

So what are you to do? Well, obviously, unless you have to work night shifts – in which case perhaps you should think about changing your job – you need to start by living your life differently and resist the temptation to stay up night after night.

Next, you should follow the detox for energy plans. If your system's become weighed down by fatigue, this will give it the kick-start it needs.

And you should also follow my seven eating tips to help keep your energy levels up to the mark at all times.

▸ Be a grazer. Eat lots of small meals throughout the day (or night) to stoke up your energy. If you don't allow yourself to get hungry, you won't reach for the high-sugar, high-fat snacks that pile on the kilos.

▸ Always carry a bag of mixed dried fruits, nuts and seeds. They'll give you a mixture of instant and slow-release energy, plus masses of vitamins and minerals.

▸ Eat as wide a variety of foods as you can. It's the easiest thing in the world to eat the same lunchtime sandwich or soup, or to take the same potato to pop in the workplace microwave, but this means that you don't get the spread of essential nutrients that you need.

▸ When winter comes, take a couple of wholemeal rolls and a thermos of high-energy hot food to work – a home-made vegetable soup, for instance, or a warming casserole or stew. Add some fresh fruit and you've got an energy-giving, sustaining and nourishing feast.

▶ Try not to eat at your desk or workstation. If there's a works canteen, there must be something healthy on the menu. If not, go out for the occasional pizza and salad or for a takeaway shish kebab in pitta bread.

▶ Pitta bread and raw vegetable sticks with a pot of hummous, guacamole or taramosalata, and a piece of exotic fresh fruit like kiwi, paw-paw or mango make an interesting energy-boosting lunchtime variation.

And when you're at work, don't forget to take proper breaks, and get some fresh air and exercise. If the weather's bad, at least find somewhere other than your desk to sit and read a paper or a book. You'll get back to work refreshed and more productive – which should please the boss!

supplementary help

You may have followed the detox programme and taken the supplements I suggested, but the following 4 are worth taking regularly. They're not meant as crutches to keep you going when you shouldn't, but they can help energize you when you need it.

▶ Guarana – the Brazilian rainforest energy herb
▶ Coenzyme Q – helps the body convert food into energy
▶ Ginseng – the Chinese herb for stamina
▶ Vitamin B complex – essential for the nervous system

kick-start your karma

In strictly chemical terms, energy is the result of combustion. The body uses the food you eat as fuel, the fuel is burnt just like the gas in your boiler, and that releases the energy that allows the body to perfom its daily tasks. But this is a very simplistic and mechanistic approach to what really happens. Since the dawn of time, shamans, medicine men, druids, priests and mystics have understood the immense power of spiritual energy and if you could learn to harness and use it yourself, you'd find a whole new dimension opening in your life. Spiritual energy will give you a reservoir of support that you can draw on whenever you need it. It will be constantly available to give the edge to the performance of whatever task you're undertaking, and you'll find that every problem is easier to resolve.

During my many years in practice, I've seen patients who eat the best possible diet and whose lives are meticulously organised, at home and at work. Yet they lack that vital spark. Life always appears to be an uphill struggle. Conversely, I've seen those who live on burgers and chips and whose lives are chaotic, but they emanate the huge vibrational force of an energetic spirit. They have an aura of stimulating and at the same time comforting and safe energy which envelops those close to them. Wherever they go, they're always the centre of attention and the reason is that they have found a way of getting in touch with their spiritual energy.

For many people, religion is the key to tapping into their spiritual energy. You may find it through formal religious belief and observance or by the loosest association with ancient mystical ideals. But it doesn't matter how you reach your goal. It's a question of what suits you best and often your personal cultural background points you in the right direction.

People tend to believe that it's only the ancient eastern religions that can take you along the path to enlightenment, but this isn't true. Certainly the traditions of the east like yoga, meditation and deep relaxation are all excellent ways to develop energy-building spiritual insights, but contrary to some misinformed opinions, it's not necessary to embrace eastern religious beliefs in order to get the benefits of meditation. You simply have to learn the physical skills necessary in order to focus your mind and concentrate on attaining a state of heightened spiritual awareness. And like all physical skills, it's simply a question of a good teacher and lots of practice.

Other people tap into their spiritual energy through the arcane arts of the druids, with their incantations and group religious ceremonies, while yet others choose a more mechanistic art, such as feng shui. Sadly, feng shui has been adopted in recent years by interior designers and so has become debased, but in fact, it's an integral part of the whole philosophy of traditional acupuncture and is dependent on a balance of yin and yang to create sensations of perfect harmony. These, in turn, bring spiritual awareness and spiritual energy.

Christianity has much to offer, too, not only for the profound beliefs it sets out, but also in terms of ritual. Using the rosary for a Catholic, contemplating icons in the Greek or Russian orthodox churches, the rituals of communion, the repetitive phrases of plainsong chant – these have exactly the same effect as Bhuddist chanting or repeating your mantra before you meditate. They're all just different ways of reaching the same goal.

I know many people whose lives have literally been turned around once they've overcome their prejudices and allowed themselves to believe that vital energy and real health come from the holistic trilogy of mind, body and spirit. But for some, this is an uncomfortable place to go. I recommend you try it – you've nothing to lose. You don't have to embrace a new religion, there is no need to give up whatever you already believe in. It can't do you any harm and for those who persevere, the rewards can be truly amazing.

shortcut to nirvana

As I've already said, relaxation exercises give your mental and emotional energy an immediate boost. This simple exercise slows the heartbeat and the breathing rate and will refresh and renew you. To begin with, you'll need about half an hour, but as you become practised, you'll reach the ideal state of mental and physical relaxation in less time.

▶ Choose a warm room, turn off the radio or television, disconnect the telephone and lie flat on a very firm bed or on a rug on the floor. Try to empty your mind of thoughts and emotions.

▶ Close your eyes and take three deep, slow breaths in and out.

▶ Stretch your left leg along the floor away from your body as hard as you can, pointing your foot and contracting the calf, thigh, buttock and lower back muscles. Hold that position until you feel a slight trembling in the muscles, then relax. Repeat with the right leg; then with both legs, and relax again.

▶ Stretch your left arm down your side, spreading your fingers and pushing from the big muscles at the back of the neck and shoulder so that you contract all the muscles of the upper arm, forearm and hand. Relax.

▶ Repeat with the right arm and relax. Repeat with both arms and relax again.

▶ Stretch both arms and legs together and relax.

▶ Take five deep breaths and repeat the cycle again. Repeat the cycle four more times.

▶ Relax totally for 10 minutes, preferably with a blanket within reach, as your body temperature may drop as a result of your slower heart beat and lower breathing rates.

the benefits of relaxation

Once you're relaxed, a number of physical and physiological changes occur within your body. You'll feel a sensation of heaviness together with a sense of clearer perception and heightened awareness. Your pulse rate will go down and because your heart is pumping more slowly, you'll be aware that your entire system seems to be slowing down too. One of the damaging effects of stress is that the levels of sugar and fat circulating in your bloodstream increase. As you become more practised at controlling your stress levels through relaxation, these levels will drop.

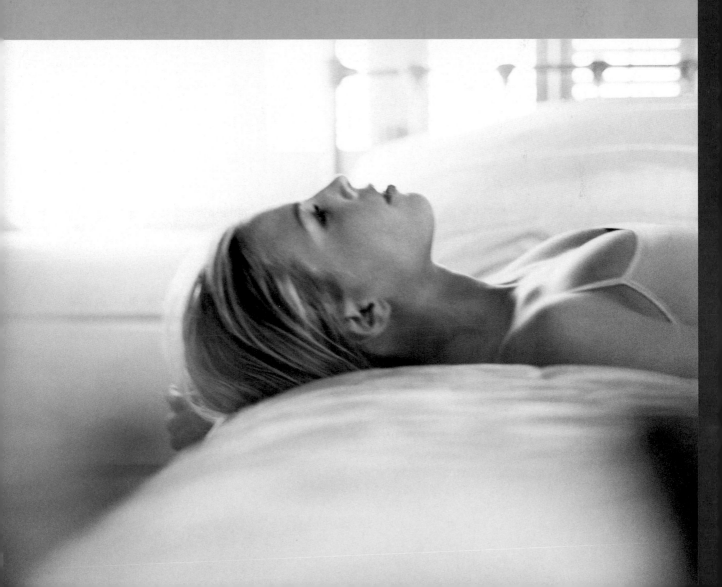

meditation

Meditation has been used for thousands of years. Its purpose is the search for the harmonisation of the way things are – reality – and the way they should be – the ideal. When you meditate, you reach a state of awareness where your mind is emptied of everything. You experience a state of restful alertness and mental and spiritual energy.

Due to its association with eastern religions, there are some fundamentalist Christians who regard all forms of meditation with suspicion. They fear that by emptying the mind you risk allowing the devil to enter it. But in fact meditation in one form or another is an integral part of many religions including Christianity. Focussing your attention on an icon in an Orthodox church, saying the rosary in a Catholic service, or concentrating on the Mandala in Tibetan Buddhism are all types of meditation.

The main components of meditation are:

▶ a clearer understanding and appreciation of the ideal order of things through enhanced awareness
▶ development of an open mind that will be receptive to reality
▶ to be spiritually and physically active in translating the ideal to reality.

The practice of meditation in the west has tended to put greatest emphasis on the understanding and appreciation of the ideal. This is visualised during periods of silent contemplation and restful alertness. To reach this state, you must focus all your concentration on a single object and to help you do this, you may constantly repeat a word or phrase, traditionally known as a mantra. This rhythmic chanting, with its hypnotic and vibrational effects, produces a trance-like state that leads your body and mind into the meditative state. It is this that produces the extraordinary health benefits. As well as producing an explosion of mental energy, regular meditation dramatically reduces your risks of heart disease, high blood pressure and strokes, and also helps combat tension, anxiety and stress-related diseases.

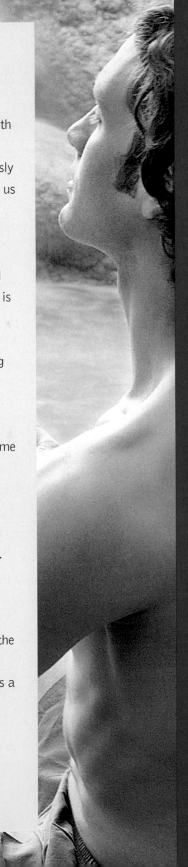

a simple guide to meditation

Over the years I've been regularly amazed at the inner peace and calm, together with the vibrant energy that I've seen in practising Buddhists and others who use meditation in their everyday lives. Experience has taught me that to become seriously involved in meditation takes the time, dedication and commitment, which not all of us are lucky enough to have. For this reason, I've devised a simplified scheme to encourage people to dip their toe into the water of this intensely spiritual practice.

If you persevere, I'm certain that you will gain so much from meditation that you'll want to understand it better and look further into its deeper meaning. Here though is where to start.

▶ Get into a comfortable position. It doesn't matter if you sit, lie or recline, as long as the radio and television are off, and you've unplugged the telephone.
▶ Close your eyes.
▶ Work your way through the Short Cut to Nirvana programme (pages 66–67).
▶ Breathe in deeply through your nose and out through your mouth, at the same time trying to empty your mind of all thoughts. While doing this, repeat your chosen mantra – the word 'one' is widely used – preferably out loud and as deeply in your voice register as you can, as this helps to create the vibration.
▶ Continue breathing deeply and evenly for at least 10 or preferably 20 minutes. Keep pushing away any distracting thoughts while constantly repeating the mantra.
▶ When you've finished, remain completely still with your eyes closed for 2–3 minutes, then open your eyes but stay where you are for another minute or two.

Deep meditation can often trigger unexpected results. Most commonly, these take the form of sudden uncontrolled emotional outbursts like laughing or crying. If this happens to you, don't worry. It's quite normal. In fact, you should be pleased as it's a sign that you really have reached a deep state of relaxation.

mind games

You've energized your body with a detox and with exercise, but your mind needs energizing as much as your body. In fact, the old adage 'use it or lose it' is just as applicable to mental processes as it is to your back, leg or any other muscles.

Of course you use your mind all day long as you make minute-to-minute decisions – you use it when you cook, shop, drive your car, even to make sure you get on the right bus. But these are hardly intellectually demanding activities and they don't stretch your mental powers.

To really generate revitalizing mental energy you have to make your brain cells work, and work hard at that. You'll only achieve this by constantly challenging your mental abilities and always seeking to push a little beyond what you think you can achieve.

improving short-term memory

Maintaining and improving short-term memory is fundamental to exercising your mental functions and allowing you to access your huge reserves of mental energy. Nothing burns up mental energy more than constantly searching through your mind for that elusive word, name, date or telephone number. Although short-term memory tends to decrease with age, it's frequently a problem of young people as well. As long as you're not suffering from any severe deterioration in brain function, every one of you should be able to sharpen up your memory and speed the access to your brain's databanks. Try the following:

▶ Kim's Game – an old stand-by of the worldwide Boy Scout movement – is one of the great memory improvers. Have someone place 20 different objects on a tray, cover it with a cloth and then allow you to look at the objects for 60 seconds. Replace the cloth, then try and write down as many objects as you can remember. Initially you may struggle to remember more than a handful, but with regular practice you'll be amazed at how quickly you'll be able to recall almost all of them.

▶ Learning by heart – you can improve both short- and long-term memory by learning poetry, speeches from plays, or quotations from well-known books. To make this work, you have to do it on a regular basis, so every night before you go to bed, commit a few lines to memory and make sure you can repeat them the next morning, and the morning after that, and a month after that. You may not have tried to memorise a poem since your schooldays, but the mental energy it generates will mean a permanent improvement. You may find you can't manage more than five or six lines to begin with but before you know it, your party piece will be the opening prologue from Shakespeare's Henry V.

exercise those brain cells

Another really effective way to prevent a decline in your short-term memory function is to practise mental arithmetic for a few minutes every single day. Try these mental maths exercises. The answers are on page 108.

1. 10 x 10 + 12

2. $\dfrac{7 \times 8 \times 2 - 2}{10}$

3. $\dfrac{13 + 7}{5 \times 12}$

4. $\dfrac{23 \times 4 - 50}{7}$

5. 17 + 14 + 106 + 33 - 27

6. 109 + 72 + 226 + 593

7. 10,425 + 8,659 + 28,694 x 100

Anagrams

1. PARTIAL MEN
2. OLD WEST ACTION
3. GENTLEMAN RYE
4. DE PEG SURREY EX NOT
5. DUESOX
6. BEG FREE RUB
7. IMBO RIN GRANTS

beat the sugar trap

Have you ever tucked into a couple of biscuits, a bowl of cornflakes or a chocolate bar? I bet you have. If so, you may have noticed how, a little while later, you feel full of pep and a few hours after that, you're jittery, unable to concentrate and dying for a little sugary fix. This is because you're now suffering – if only in passing – from hypoglaecaemia or low blood-sugar. It's sometimes called the 'Sugar Blues'.

When carbohydrate foods are eaten, the sugars they contain are broken down into glucose during digestion. Glucose – or blood sugar as it is also confusingly known – is the fuel our bodies run on. The glucose circulating in our bloodstream after a carbohydrate meal is circulated to cells for instant use, and any surplus is converted into glycogen and stored as fuel in the liver, ready to be 'switched on' whenever it is needed. The hormone insulin, secreted by the pancreas, is responsible for this storage job.

Eat a slice of wholegrain bread, a dish of lentils, or a handful of ripe apricots, and the sugars in them are broken down into glucose quite slowly. But when you eat your biscuits, cornflakes or chocolate – known as high-glycaemic foods – the sugars they contain will be broken down very quickly, sending the glucose level in your bloodstream rocketing.

The pancreas responds to this abnormal situation by pumping out extra insulin, so your blood-sugar levels drop sharply – giving you the 'Sugar Blues'.

The sugar in processed food – aided and abetted by the food-manufacturing industry – is obviously the real villain of the piece and it's hard to avoid. It's there in desserts, juices, canned drinks, sugar-coated breakfast cereals, biscuits, ice cream, snacks and sweets. Once you've acquired a sweet tooth, it's not long before every cup of tea or coffee needs three heaped spoons of sugar and every unoccupied moment is filled with a biscuit, a piece of cake, or a Danish pastry.

the effects on your health

The fluctuations in blood-sugar levels caused by eating these foods have been linked with a huge spectrum of health problems. Long-term, they will be responsible for high blood pressure, obesity, diabetes and heart disease. In children they may be responsible for disruptive behaviour, hyperactivity and an inability to concentrate. And one of the commonest symptoms of low blood sugar is mental and physical fatigue – which may account for the state of permanent exhaustion suffered by so many adults, teenagers and children.

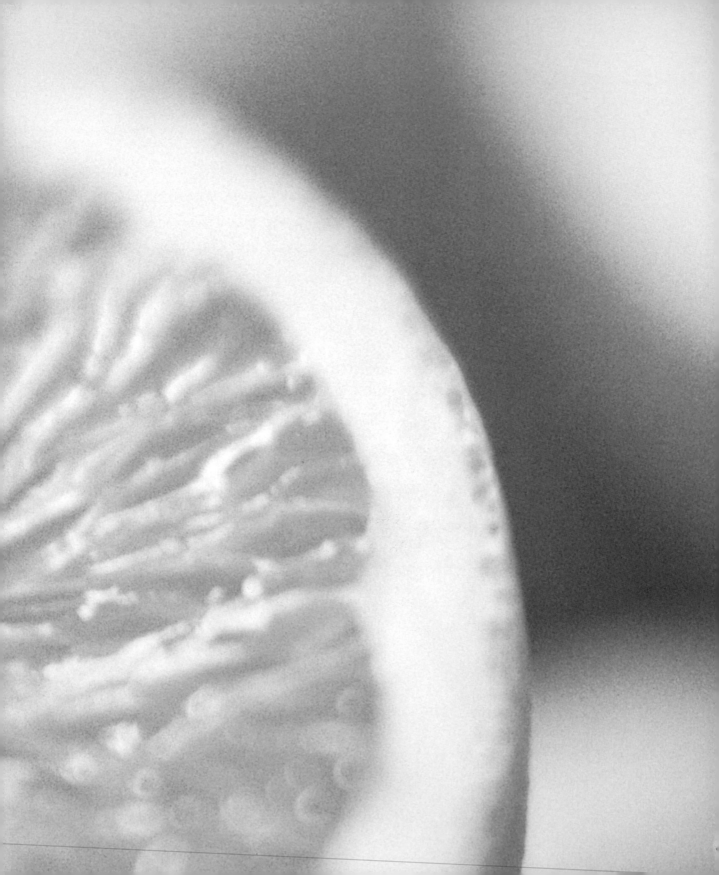

the glycaemic index

The glycaemic index – GI – is a way of calculating the rate at which carbohydrate foods are digested and converted into sugar by the body. The lower a food's GI, the longer it takes for that food to be converted into sugar. Using the GI can be a great help in planning a healthy diet that will provide you with a gradual release of energy and so help you avoid the sugar trap. By mixing low GI foods into a meal, you'll be able to maintain a much more even level of blood sugar and so ensure a constant flow of mental and physical energy.

Taking 100 as the standard, processed foods like white bread, sugared breakfast cereals, puffed rice, cornflakes, puffed wheat, sweet biscuits, instant mashed potato, corn chips, and glucose and honey, all have a GI between 70 and 100. Foods with a GI below 60 are wholemeal wheat, rye and pumpernickel, wholemeal pasta, brown rice, sweetcorn, buckwheat, bulgur, wholewheat kernels, whole rye kernels, pearl barley, shredded wheat, oatmeal, chickpeas, soya beans, all dried beans, and low-fat dairy foods.

other processed-food problems

While we all need plenty of carbohydrate foods to give us physical as well as mental energy, the best of them supply more than just energy. Foods such as wholegrain bread, brown rice, whole oats, beans and lentils and fruits are also loaded with important nutrients and are rich in fibre which helps keep the digestive system functioning efficiently. But when these foods are refined or heavily processed, they lose not only a whole slew of vital nutrients, but most of the fibre too.

To take just one example, white flour contains much less zinc (essential for resistance, mental energy and male sexual function), much less magnesium (vital for the nervous system and also for the absorption of calcium), and significantly less protein (essential for body-building) than wholemeal flour. Token amounts of major nutrients are added back when white flour is baked into bread, but not when it goes into other foods.

It's the same story when rice and maize are refined. And white sugar has absolutely no nutritional value at all, except for a lot of energy-giving calories – styled 'empty' calories for this very reason. Brown sugar and honey at least contain traces of key nutrients.

some real life stories

The sugar trap can affect anyone, regardless of age, occupation or social status. Once you're in the trap, it's hard to get out unless you know how. More often than not, it's life's circumstances that create the eating patterns that lead you into the trap, rather than the deliberate adoption of dreadful eating habits.

the concert pianist's story

One of the world's leading concert pianists came to see me suffering from ever-increasing fatigue, irritabiltity and memory and concentration problems. He'd done the round of doctors and tests and had ended up being prescribed anti-depressants, but wasn't happy to take them.

His problems were all the result of his lifestyle. He couldn't eat a proper meal before a performance, so used high-sugar snacks to give him the energy to play. After concerts there were always parties with junk food and alcohol and the next morning he would have a hangover, so couldn't eat breakfast. He got through his day's practising with endless cups of sweet tea, coffee, biscuits and chocolate. No wonder his blood-sugar levels were like a yo-yo. And added to that was endless travel, airline meals, jetlag and hotel food.

The first step was to turn him into a 'grazer', eating little but often. He needed to avoid all alcohol for a month and drink a maximum of 6 cups a day of tea and coffee, halving the sugar he took each week until he wasn't taking any at all.

I gave him an eating plan. Breakfast was essential – he needed a combination of protein and complex carbohydrate, so I suggested baked beans on toast, a bowl of porridge or muesli with fresh fruit or 2 eggs, wholemeal toast and a small piece of cheese. He was allowed a handful of mixed fresh unsalted, unroasted nuts, seeds and dried fruit every hour, a banana in the middle of the morning and another mid-afternoon.

Lunch time was a protein and starch mix again – pasta with a cheese- or meat-based sauce or salad with fish, meat or poultry, and mid-afternoon he was also allowed a small portion of muesli. Before the perfomance he could have a very light snack such as scrambled eggs, a tuna or bean salad, or an easily digested sandwich, and he could have a handful of nuts, seeds and raisins during the interval and a couple more again at the end of the concert.

Within six weeks, he was back to his normal, energetic and vibrant self!

the social worker's story

Miss A was a social worker who came to see me. 'Whenever my colleagues and I caught flu, they got better but I got worse. From being a bubbly, extrovert, I found myself at home crying. I hoped I'd had my share of health problems as I'd suffered one illness after another from childhood till my teens. But it was the flu that floored me. I was so ill, I didn't work for six months, then soon after I went back, I got ill again and my doctor diagnosed ME.

'I didn't work for the next four years but I was lucky enough to finally get a less demanding job. I now work 36 hours a week, but on bad days I can take time off and make it up later. It's the lack of energy that really worries me. I take my dog to training classes and there are 70-year-olds more energetic than I am! And because I'm always so tired, I can't be active and I'm now 25 kilos overweight.'

This was such a typical story. ME is devastating, but Miss A needed to help herself. Her daily diet consisted of muesli with goat's milk, wholemeal toast and marmalade, tea with goat's milk, bread and honey, banana, coffee, curry and brown rice. This is low in calcium and vitamin D (both essential for bones), low in B vitamins (vital for the nervous system and energy creation), very short of iodine (for the thyroid), and she got a quarter of all her calories from sugar.

Worst of all was her weight. She was carrying 300 quarter-kilo packets of lard, which was perhaps a worse problem than the ME. She needed exercise – a 10-minute walk three times a day for starters – and to eat lots more oily fish. She also needed more low-GI foods like oats, brown rice, wholemeal bread and beans and pasta, and much less sugar. Like the pianist, I recommended that she become a grazer and eat at least five small meals a day. This would give her a constant supply of blood sugar and so help maintain her physical and mental energy. And I also suggested she take a B-complex pill, kelp and guarana. These would make a huge difference too.

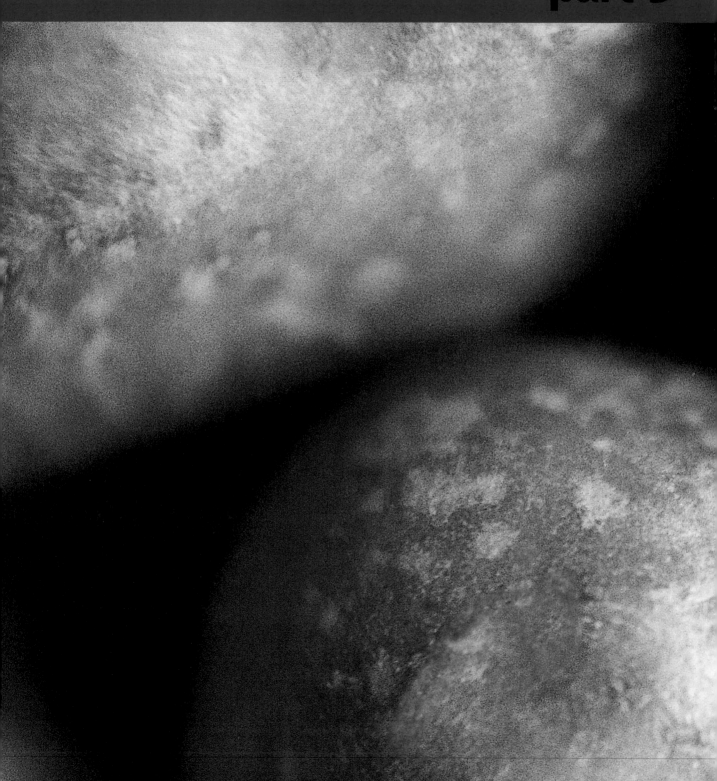

eat your way to super energy

all recipes serve 4, except drinks recipes which serve 2

bread and breakfast

energy teabread

Earl Grey tea	300ml, made with 5 teabags and left to cool
dried dates	450g, chopped into raisin-sized pieces
demerara sugar	200g
egg	1, beaten
self-raising flour	250g

People often think treats like this are sinful, but this certainly isn't. One generous slice will be a huge boost to your flagging energy, and thanks to the dates, provides iron, fibre and plenty of disease-fighting antioxidants.

Mix all the ingredients together and leave to stand, covered with a clean tea towel, for at least 6 hours. Preheat the oven to 180°C/350°F/Gas 4. Pour into a 1.2 litre loaf tin lined with greaseproof paper. Bake in the preheated oven for 30 minutes. Turn out of the tin and leave to cool on a wire rack.

real swiss muesli

organic, low-salt, unsweetened muesli	12 heaped tbsp,
apple juice	about 500ml
live natural yoghurt	about 500g

The slow-release energy from the oats makes them perfect for breakfast or brunch as they help keep your blood sugar on an even keel for several hours. This means you avoid those mid-morning sugar cravings.

Put the muesli into 2 bowls. Pour on the apple juice – don't worry if the mixture seems very runny; the cereal will expand. Stir in the yoghurt and leave in the fridge overnight.

porridge with cinnamon and dried fruits

porridge oats	2 average cups
semi-skimmed milk	2 average cups
water	2 average cups
mixed dried fruits	150g
ground cinnamon	2 level tsp

This has all the energy and blood sugar benefits of the oats, plus the huge antioxidant and protective value of the fruits.

Put the oats, milk and water into a saucepan. Bring to the boil and simmer for 5 minutes or according to the packet instructions, stirring regularly. While it's cooking, cut the dried fruits into evenly sized pieces, about as big as a little fingernail. When the porridge is cooked, stir in the fruit and 1 tsp of cinnamon. Cover and leave to rest for 2 minutes. Serve with the remaining cinnamon sprinkled on top and extra milk, if desired.

scrambled eggs with smoked salmon

unsalted butter	50g
semi-skimmed milk	150ml
eggs	8 medium
smoked salmon	110g of trimmings – you don't need expensive slices – cut into fine slivers
black pepper	to taste
chives	10, snipped
toast or rustic bread	to serve

Put the butter and milk in a large, preferably nonstick, frying pan and heat gently until the butter has melted. Remove the pan from the heat and crack in the eggs. Gently break up the yolks, but don't amalgamate them fully with the egg white. Return to a low heat. Using a wooden spatula, push the mixture regularly from the edges to the middle of the pan, again leaving some definition between the yolks and whites. When the eggs are almost as firm as you like them – the heat of the pan will continue the cooking process for several minutes – remove the pan from the heat and stir in the smoked salmon. Season to taste with freshly ground black pepper and serve with the chives sprinkled on top and accompanied by toast or chunks of rustic bread.

mushrooms on wholemeal toast

mushrooms	300g any well-flavoured variety
unsalted butter	1150g, preferably unsalted
parsley	4 large sprigs, leaves finely chopped
wholemeal bread	4 slices, preferably organic

Wipe and slice the mushrooms. Melt the butter gently in a small frying pan and add the chopped parsley. Sauté the mushrooms over a low heat until the juices run, about 10 minutes. Just before they're cooked, toast the bread and serve with the mushroom mixture piled on top.

buckwheat crêpes

Crêpes always seem like an indulgence, but the rutin and natural chemicals in buckwheat ensure that energizing oxygen nutrients get to where they need to be and protect the tiniest blood vessels.

butter	50g
semi-skimmed milk	425ml
buckwheat flour	110g
organic plain flour	110g, sifted
salt	¼ tsp
eggs	4, medium
rapeseed oil	for frying
pumpkin seeds	50g
lemons	juice of 2 large
runny honey	4 tbsp

Melt the butter and stir it into the milk. Put the flours and salt together in a food processor. Whisking continuously, pour in the milk and butter mixture. Still whisking, add the eggs one at a time until you have a smooth batter. Leave the mixture to rest in the fridge for at least 1 hour.

Brush a crêpe pan or small frying pan with a little oil and heat over a medium heat until the oil is smoking. Pour in a ladleful of batter, tilting the pan to spread it evenly. When the underside is golden, turn the crêpe – or toss it if you feel like showing off – and cook for a further 1–2 minutes. Slide the crêpe onto kitchen paper and keep warm while you repeat with the rest of the batter.

Dry-fry the pumpkin seeds for 2 minutes, until just turning colour. Drizzle each crêpe with the lemon juice and honey, fold in half and serve with the pumpkin seeds scattered on top.

savoury toasties

unsalted butter	for spreading
wholewheat bread	4 thick slices
tomatoes	2, sliced
green pepper	½, deseeded and very finely chopped
onion	1 small, very finely chopped
paprika	2 pinches
Gruyère cheese	2 heaped tbsp, grated

Preheat the oven to 230°C/450°F/Gas 8. Butter the bread, arrange the slices of tomato on top and cook in the preheated oven for 7 minutes. Put the chopped pepper and onion on top of the tomatoes with a pinch of paprika on each slice. Sprinkle the cheese on top and return to the oven until the cheese is bubbling, about 5 minutes.

poached kippers and tomatoes

kippers	2 pairs, undyed
tomatoes	4
unsalted butter	50g
lemon	juice of ½
parsley	1 heaped tbsp finely chopped leaves

Even though kippers are salty, they're a great source of energy-producing protein and also provide some iodine, which is essential for the effective action of the thyroid. The fish oils in kippers are also an anti-inflammatory and vital for heart protection.

Bring a large shallow saucepan of water to the boil. Add the kippers and tomatoes and simmer for about 5 minutes. Meanwhile, cream the butter and stir in the lemon juice and parsley and reserve until required. Remove the kippers and tomatoes from the water with a slotted spoon. Pat the kippers dry with kitchen paper. Slip the skins off the tomatoes. Serve with a knob of the prepared butter on each kipper.

english breakfast the healthy way

mushrooms	2, large, wiped
bacon	4 extra-lean rashers
traditional sausages with a high meat content	4
tomatoes	2, halved widthways
eggs	4, medium
wholemeal bread, toasted	to serve

I'm convinced that one factor in the epidemic of chronic fatigue is people's failure to eat a proper breakfast. The traditional English breakfast has been so criticised that rather than eat it at home, many people sneak off to a café on their way to work. My old friend and first of the super chefs, Anton Mosimann, taught me the egg trick.

Preheat the grill and line a grill rack with foil. Put the mushrooms, bacon, sausages and tomatoes on the grill rack and put under the grill. While they're cooking, put a large plate on top of a saucepan of simmering water. When the plate is really hot, break the eggs onto it and leave to cook. Serve this traditional breakfast with good wholemeal toast.

drinks

In all detox plans, maintaining a high fluid intake is essential if you are to achieve the overall cleansing benefits you're aiming for. These simple recipes for juices and smoothies are specifically compiled to give you a real energy boost. They're here for two reasons: firstly, to help you cope with your reduced calorie intake during the detox programmes, and secondly, to get you into the habit of using and enjoying these high-energy and super-nutrient drinks as part of your normal life.

It's surprising how much of an energy bonus you can get from these delicious drinks. The high natural sugar content of carrots, apples, beetroot and bananas gets you off to a great start, the protein and oils in the peanuts release their energy just when the instant boost starts to run down, and the more complex starches in the banana are also a good supply of slower-release energy with lots of potassium for sustained activity if you're sporty.

carrot, apple and beetroot juice

carrots	3, large, topped and tailed – and peeled if not organic
apples	2, quartered
beetroot	2, small, raw with leaves

It's the high natural sugar content of the beetroot that makes this juice an energy booster. But there's an added bonus in the form of the skin-friendly vitamin A in the carrots.

Simply put all the ingredients in a blender or liquidizer and whizz together until smooth.

carrot, apple and celery juice

carrots	3, large, topped and tailed – and peeled if not organic
apples	2, quartered
celery	2 stalks

Simply put all the ingredients in a blender or liquidizer and whizz together until smooth.

yoghurt and fruit smoothie

live natural yoghurt	500g
strawberries	600g
coriander	6 large stalks

Simply put all the ingredients in a blender or liquidizer and whizz together until smooth.

apple, peanut and banana smoothie

apples	3, quartered and juiced
bananas	2
peanut butter	2 tbsp, smooth
soya milk	500ml

An excellent start to anybody's day thanks to the high-energy value of the bananas and peanuts. This smoothie also provides the health benefits of soya milk, which helps protect against hormonal swings, osteoporosis and breast cancer.

Simply put all the ingredients in a blender or liquidizer and whizz together until smooth.

mango, kiwi and pineapple juice

mango	1, large, ripe stoned
kiwi fruit	4
pineapple	1, medium, top removed

Simply put all the ingredients in a blender or liquidizer and whizz together until smooth.

lunches and dinners

mediterranean omelette flan

ready-rolled puff pastry	1 sheet
garlic	3 cloves, finely chopped
tomatoes	200g, deseeded and roughly chopped
stoned olives	110g, rinsed and halved
parsley, chervil, oregano and chives	5 tbsp freshly chopped leaves
live natural yoghurt	200g
eggs	4

Preheat the oven to 220°C/425°F/Gas 7. Use the pastry to line a 29 x 20cm loose-bottomed flan tin. Scatter the garlic, tomatoes and olives over the pastry and sprinkle over the herbs. Mix together the yoghurt and eggs and pour over the filling. Bake in the preheated oven for 30 minutes.

large grilled prawns on salad leaves
This recipe works excellently on a barbecue.

Pacific prawns (or other large variety with shells)	20
garlic	5 cloves, finely chopped
extra-virgin olive oil	100ml
mixed salad leaves	1 large packet
lemons	2, halved

Wash the prawns under cold running water and dry thoroughly with kitchen paper. Mix together the garlic and olive oil in a large bowl. Add the prawns and stir to coat thoroughly. Cover with clingfilm and leave to marinate in the fridge for 2 hours. Preheat the grill to high. Remove the prawns from the marinade with a slotted spoon and cook under the preheated grill, basting with the marinade until the shells are almost burned, about 4 minutes on each side. Serve on a bed of salad leaves, with lemon halves to squeeze over.

green pasta with tuna fish

spinach tagliatelle	450g
extra-virgin olive oil	2 tbsp
spring onions	4, large, chopped (including the green parts)
tuna	1 x 400g can
tomatoes	4, large, roughly chopped

Cook the pasta in a large saucepan of boiling water according to the packet instructions. Meanwhile, heat the oil in a saucepan and sauté the spring onions gently until soft. Add the tuna and warm through gently. Drain the pasta and return to the pan. Mix the fish and onion mixture, with the tomatoes, into the pasta and serve.

dutch chicken

basmati rice	350g
sesame oil	3 tbsp
chicken breasts	450g skinless, cut into slivers along the grain
carrot	1, very thinly sliced
green pepper	1, deseeded, very thinly sliced
Chinese five-spice powder or allspice	3 tsp
fresh root ginger	2.5cm, peeled and grated
soy sauce	3 tbsp
fresh beansprouts	225g
spring onions	5, trimmed and finely sliced on the diagonal

The Dutch were the first to bring Indonesian cuisine to Europe, hence the name of this recipe. In it, the combination of chicken and rice provides protein and an enormous amount of energy. The vegetables add a nutritional bonus, while the Oriental flavour of the spices makes this dish really special.

Cook the rice in a saucepan of boiling water according to the packet instructions. Meanwhile, heat the oil in a preheated wok or large frying pan and stir-fry the chicken for 5 minutes. Add the carrot and green pepper and continue cooking for a further 2 minutes. Add the spices and soy sauce and stir well. Add the rest of the ingredients, including the drained rice, and cook for a further 3 minutes, still stirring vigorously.

pasta all'aglio e olio

spaghettini	400g
extra-virgin olive oil	6 tbsp
garlic	3 cloves, peeled and crushed with the flat blade of a broad knife
Parmesan cheese	4 tbsp, freshly grated
fresh basil	6 large sprigs, leaves removed and finely torn

This recipe is just as good for your health as it is for boosting your energy. It's an excellent source of slow-release calories, which provide a sustained increase in energy levels for two to three hours. The health-giving fats in the olive oil take even longer to convert to useable energy, so you get an extra spurt just when you've used up the energy provided by the pasta.

Cook the pasta according to the packet instructions. Meanwhile, heat the olive oil in a saucepan, add the garlic and cook gently until just beginning to turn brown. Remove the garlic with a slotted spoon and discard. Pour the hot oil over the pasta and mix thoroughly. Stir in the Parmesan cheese and mix again. Finally, stir in the basil leaves and serve immediately.

spanish omelette

extra-virgin olive oil	3 tbsp
potatoes	4, small, new, unpeeled and cubed
red pepper	1, small, diced
onion	1, sliced
courgettes	2, small, diced
eggs	6
dried mixed herbs	1 tsp

The versatility of this high-energy protein dish is that it's as good hot as it is cold. You can serve it for breakfast, lunch or supper. The vegetables provide masses of nutrients to accompany the energy-giving potatoes.

Warm the olive oil in a large frying pan. Add the potatoes and stir until just turning golden. Add the peppers and onions and stir for 2 minutes until soft. Add the courgettes and stir for a further 1 minute. Beat the eggs and mix in the dried herbs. Pour the egg mixture into the pan and cook until set. Depending on how large your pan is, you may need to finish off cooking the omelette under a hot preheated grill.

italian toast

coarse wholemeal bread	4 thick slices
garlic	2 plump cloves, halved
extra-virgin olive oil	about 4 tbsp
avocado	1 large or 2 small, mashed just before use
tomatoes	2, large, thinly sliced
Parma ham	2 slices
mozzarella cheese	1 small packet, sliced

Perfect for a Sunday morning brunch. Lots of energy from the bread, protein from the ham and cheese, plus calcium, vitamin E and all the protective nutrients in the garlic, avocados and tomatoes.

Preheat the grill and line a grill rack with foil. Toast the bread until just golden on both sides. Rub one side of each slice with the cut side of garlic. Drizzle on a little of the olive oil. Spread the avocado on top, followed by the slices of tomato, Parma ham and mozzarella cheese. Cook under the preheated grill until the cheese is just melted.

gratin of potatoes and mushrooms

butter	50g
potatoes	450g, peeled and thinly sliced
mushrooms	225g, wiped and finely sliced
salt and pepper	to season
basic stock (see recipe, page 96)	75ml
single cream	75ml
garlic	2 cloves, very finely chopped

Preheat the oven to 180°C/350°F/Gas 4. Use half the butter to grease a shallow casserole. Arrange the potatoes and mushrooms in alternating layers, seasoning with salt and pepper as you go and finishing with the potatoes. Mix together the stock and cream and pour onto the dish. Dot the rest of the butter and the garlic over the top. Cover with foil and bake in the preheated oven for 1 hour. Remove the foil and leave the dish in the oven for a further 10 minutes until the potatoes are golden.

millet and mushroom risotto

extra-virgin olive oil	3 tbsp
onion	1, large, finely chopped
garlic	2 large cloves, finely chopped
millet	250g
green pepper	1, diced
basic stock (see recipe, page 96)	850ml
bouquet garni	1
bay leaves	2
mushrooms	275g, wiped and sliced

Delicious as a brunch, this recipe combines slow-release energy from the millet, vitamin C from the pepper and the immune-boosting properties of onions, mushrooms and garlic.

Heat the oil in a large saucepan, add the onion and sweat until soft. Add the garlic and cook for 1 minute. Add the millet and stir for 2 minutes. Add the green pepper and cook for a further 2 minutes. Add the stock, bouquet garni and bay leaves, cover the pan and simmer gently for 15 minutes. Stir in the mushrooms and continue cooking for 5 minutes. Remove the bouquet garni and bay leaves before serving.

chillied sardine sandwiches

sardines	2 x 100g cans in olive oil
Worcestershire sauce	1 tbsp
lemon	juice of ½
wholemeal bread	4 thick slices

Mix the sardines, including the oil, with the Worcestershire sauce and lemon. Pile the mixture onto the bread and serve.

non-meatballs in tomato sauce

vegeburger mix	450g
garlic	3 cloves, finely chopped
mint	2 tbsp freshly chopped leaves
parsley	2 tbsp freshly chopped leaves
tomatoes	1 x 400g can
vegetable stock cube	1
white wine	4 tbsp
onion	1, large, finely chopped
extra-virgin olive oil	1 tbsp
green chilli	1, deseeded and finely chopped
rapeseed oil	100ml

Prepare the vegeburger mix according to the packet instructions, adding the garlic, mint and parsley. Put the tomatoes and their juice into a large frying pan with the crumbled stock cube, wine, onion, olive oil and chilli. Bring to the boil and simmer for 10 minutes. While the sauce is cooking, form the vegeburger mixture into walnut-sized balls and fry gently in the rapeseed oil for 3 minutes on each side. Add them to the tomato sauce and serve immediately.

spiced chickpea casserole

rapeseed oil	4 tbsp
onions	2, sliced
aubergine	1, sliced
peppers	1 red, 1 yellow, 1 green, deseeded and sliced into rings
potatoes	2, large, peeled and sliced
chickpeas	1 x 400g can, drained and rinsed
garlic	2 cloves, finely chopped
paprika	1 tsp
allspice	1 tsp
olive paste	2 tsp
tomatoe purée	2 tsp
very veggie stock (see recipe, page 97)	450ml
chopped tomatoes	1 x 200g can

Preheat the oven to 190°C/375°F/Gas 5. Heat the oil in a frying pan and sauté the onions until soft. Remove and set aside on kitchen paper to remove the excess oil. Using the same oil, adding more if necessary, repeat with the aubergines and peppers. Layer the vegetables and chickpeas in a casserole dish. Sprinkle over the garlic, paprika and allspice. Mix together the olive paste, tomato purée and 2 tbsp of water and pour over the casserole. Mix together the stock and tomatoes and pour over the dish, adding enough water to almost cover. Cover and cook in the preheated oven for 90 minutes.

spicy energy beans

unsalted butter	25g
onion	1, medium, finely chopped
garlic	2 cloves, finely chopped
paprika	1 tsp
kidney beans	2 x 400g cans, rinsed and drained
very veggie stock (see recipe, page 97)	600ml
coriander	2 tbsp freshly chopped leaves
garam masala	1 tbsp
cooked rice	to serve

Heat the butter in a saucepan and sauté the onions gently until soft. Add the garlic and paprika. Stir thoroughly and cook over a medium heat, stirring continuously, for 2 minutes. Add the beans, stock, coriander and garam masala. Cover and simmer for 5 minutes. Serve with rice.

steak in red wine

fillet steaks	4, about 2.5cm thick
plain flour	4 tbsp
rapeseed oil	2 tbsp
unsalted butter	25g
garlic	2 cloves, finely chopped
full-bodied red wine, such as Chianti or Barolo	250ml
salt and pepper	to season

Dust the steaks with the flour. Heat the oil and butter in a large frying pan until the butter stops foaming. Add the garlic, then add the steaks and cook for 1 minute on each side. Remove the steaks and reserve until required. Pour in the wine and simmer, stirring continuously, until reduced by half. Season the steaks with salt and pepper, return to the pan and cook for 2–3 minutes each side, depending on how rare you like them. Serve immediately.

baked cod with sesame seeds

cod steaks	4
eggs	2, beaten
sesame seeds	110g

It's the energy boost from the sesame seeds that makes this simple dish different. Like all seeds, sesame seeds are rich in vitamin E.

Preheat the oven to 170°C/325°F/Gas 3. Dip the fish into the eggs, then the sesame seeds. Put on a large baking sheet and cook in the preheated oven for 20 minutes.

beef stir-fry

rump steak	400g, fat removed and cut into thin strips
cornflour	1 tbsp
Chinese five-spice powder	¼ tsp
light soy sauce	4 tbsp
sesame oil	4 tbsp
fresh root ginger	2.5cm, peeled and grated
garlic	2 cloves, finely chopped
green pepper	1, small, deseeded and cubed
broccoli	175g very small florets, stems cut finely on the diagonal
spring onions	6, trimmed and cut on the diagonal
dry sherry	4 tbsp
rice or noodles	to serve

Put the meat into a large bowl with the thoroughly mixed cornflour, spice and soy sauce. Cover and leave to marinate in the fridge for 30 minutes, then drain. Heat the oil in a preheated wok or large frying pan, add the steak, ginger and garlic and stir-fry for 4 minutes. Add the pepper, broccoli and spring onions and continue cooking for 2 minutes. Pour in the sherry and 2 tbsp of water, cover and leave to steam for 1 minute. Serve with rice or noodles.

lamb and pine-kernel koftas

wooden skewers	4
onion	1, coarsely chopped
pine kernels	50g
lamb mince	450g, fresh, or the minced leftovers from Sunday lunch
mint	2 tbsp freshly chopped leaves
egg	1
pitta bread	to serve
green salad	to serve

Soak the skewers in water for 30 minutes before using to prevent burning. Preheat the grill and line a grill rack with foil. Put the onion and pine kernels into a food processor or blender and chop finely. Add the lamb, mint and egg and blend to a smoothish purée. Mould into walnut-sized balls and thread onto kebab sticks. Grill under the preheated grill for 2 minutes on each side. Serve with pitta bread and a green salad.

ten-minute mussels

unsalted butter	50g
shallots	4, very finely chopped
garlic	very finely chopped
red chilli	1, deseeded and finely chopped
parsley	5 tbsp freshly chopped leaves
dry white wine	½ bottle
mussels	2kg, washed, beards removed and any open shells discarded

Melt the butter in a pan large enough to hold all the mussels and sauté the shallots, garlic and chilli gently. Add the chopped parsley, pour in the wine and bring to the boil. Add the mussels. Cover the pan and cook over a medium heat for 5 minutes until the shells open. Discard any that don't open. Using a slotted spoon, put the mussels into serving bowls. Bring the rest of the liquid to a very fast boil for 3 minutes. Pour over the mussels and serve.

squash, almond and raisin bulgur

bulgur	150g
olive oil	at least 6 tbsp
onions	2, large, very finely sliced
squash or courgettes	350g, peeled, deseeded and cubed
ground coriander	12 tsp
ground cumin	12 tsp
flaked almonds	150g
raisins	110g
salt and black pepper	to season

This energy-giving vegetable dish is another fast/slow energy meal thanks to the fruit, the sugar and the grains. If you've never cooked with bulgur before, do try this recipe. It's a wonderful wheat and cooking it is as easy as cooking rice.

Simmer the bulgur in twice its volume of water for 10 minutes until most of the water is absorbed. Meanwhile, heat 2 tbsp of the oil and fry the onion until it is brown but not crisp. Add the squash and sauté until brown, adding more oil if necessary. Sprinkle in the spices and cook for 1 minute, stirring continuously. Reduce the heat, add the almonds and raisins and continue cooking, still stirring, until the almonds are golden. Drain the bulgur, if necessary, and stir into the vegetable mixture. Season to taste with salt and black pepper. Add more oil if the mixture looks too dry and heat through for 1 minute.

posh cauliflower cheese with pasta

sun-dried tomatoes	275g
spaghetti	
cauliflower	1, cut into small florets
extra-virgin olive oil	4 tbsp
onion	1, large, finely chopped
dry white wine	75ml
eggs	2, beaten
Parmesan cheese	3 tbsp, freshly grated
fresh basil	4 tbsp roughly torn leaves

The pasta, oil and cheese in this different type of traditional cauliflower cheese give you masses of energy. And as a bonus, there's the calcium in the cheese and plenty of cancer-protective nutrients in the cauliflower.

Cook the pasta according to the instructions on the packet. Meanwhile, blanch the cauliflower in boiling water for 2 minutes, then drain. Heat the olive oil in a large saucepan and sauté the onion gently. Add the cauliflower and wine and simmer gently. Mix together the eggs, cheese and half the basil. Drain the cooked pasta and add to the cauliflower. Pour over the egg mixture, stirring continuously over a gentle heat until the egg scrambles. Sprinkle over the extra basil leaves and serve.

grilled lamb cutlets with rosemary

lamb cutlets	4
extra-virgin olive oil	6 tbsp
garlic	2 cloves, finely chopped
fresh rosemary	4 tbsp very finely chopped leaves

Trim any excess fat off the cutlets. Mix the oil, garlic and rosemary together in a large shallow dish. Add the cutlets and turn to coat in the marinade. Cover and leave to marinate in the fridge for 2 hours, turning occasionally. Preheat the grill to high. Remove the cutlets from the marinade, leaving some of the liquid still clinging, and cook under the preheated grill for 2–3 minutes on each side. Serve immediately.

brown rice risotto with sun-dried tomatoes

rapeseed oil	3 tbsp
onion	1, finely chopped
garlic	2 cloves, finely chopped
brown rice	225g
sun-dried tomatoes	200g
tomatoes	4, roughly chopped
very veggie stock (see recipe, page 97)	800ml
Cheddar cheese	3 tbsp, grated
basil	10 leaves, roughly torn

Strictly speaking, you cook risotto by stirring the stock in gradually over about 30 minutes. But this dish is more of a boiled rice with vegetables than a risotto. It's easier, extremely high in energy and delicious hot or cold.

Heat the oil in a large non-stick frying pan and sauté the onion and garlic gently until just turning golden. Add the rice, sun-dried tomatoes snipped to the size of a raisin, fresh tomatoes and stock. Simmer for 40 minutes, adding extra stock or water, if necessary. Stir in the cheese, sprinkle on the basil and serve.

duck breasts with pepper sauce

unsalted butter	50g
duck breasts	4, skinless
onion	1, finely chopped
green peppercorns	2 tbsp
red wine	100ml
crème fraîche	4 tbsp

Heat the butter in a large frying pan and sauté the duck breasts for about 4 minutes until they are golden. Remove and keep warm. Add the onion to the pan and sauté until golden. Add the peppercorns and red wine and simmer for 10 minutes. Add the crème fraîche and continue to simmer for 3 minutes. Meanwhile, slice the duck breasts diagonally and arrange on the serving plates. Pour over the peppercorn sauce and serve.

grilled italian vegetables

courgettes	4, small, halved lengthways
aubergine	1, large, sliced widthways
peppers	1 red, 1 yellow, deseeded and cut into wide strips
extra-virgin olive oil	5 tbsp
Little Gem lettuces	2, broken into leaves
mushroom	1, large, field variety, wiped and quartered
garlic	2 cloves, finely chopped
mozzarella	1 piece, sliced

Preheat the grill and line the grill pan with foil. Add the vegetables and brush with half the olive oil. Cook for 3 minutes on each side. Put the lettuce onto an ovenproof plate and place the mushroom quarters on top. Arrange the grilled vegetables over the whole dish, then drizzle over the rest of the oil and sprinkle over the garlic. Top with the mozzarella slices and return to the hot grill for 1 minute or until the cheese has melted.

roman liver

sage leaves	16
sunflower oil	4 tbsp
unsalted butter	50g
calves' liver	8 thin slices, weighing about 500g in total
limes	2, halved, to serve

Fry the sage leaves in the oil for 1 minute until crisp. Remove with a slotted spoon and drain on kitchen paper. Wipe the pan and add the butter. Heat until foaming, add the liver slices and cook for 1 minute on each side. Serve with the sage leaves on top and the lime halves on the side.

soups and salads

Here I start with three basic stock and salad dressing recipes that are the result of my many years of helping develop optimum diets for my patients. Making your own stocks and dressings guarantees that you avoid the energy-sapping, anti-nutrient chemicals in nearly all commercial products and that you consume only fresh, natural micro-nutrients.

basic chicken stock

chicken	1 carcass – the remains of the Sunday roast will do, but it's better to ask a butcher to keep a carcass which has been stripped of its other useful meat.
water	2 litres
spring onions	6, with the stalks on
leeks	1, large, trimmed and coarsely chopped
celery	2 large stalks, chopped
rosemary	1 large sprig
parsley	2 generous handfuls
sage	1 large sprig
thyme	2 large sprigs
bay leaves	3
white peppercorns	10

Put the chicken carcass into a large heavy-based saucepan and cover with the water. Bring to the boil and cook, uncovered, for 30 minutes. Add the rest of the ingredients, partially cover the pan and simmer for 40 minutes, adding more water if necessary. Strain and use as required.

very veggie stock

onions	2; 1 peeled and quartered, 1 left whole
celery	3 large stalks, with their leaves
leeks	1
parsnip	1
sage	1 large sprig
thyme	2 sprigs
bay leaves	6
parsley	2 generous handfuls
black peppercorns	12
water	2 litres

This basic recipe may seem as if it takes a long time and will leave you with far more stock that you need. But it's simple to make and healthier than any commercial stock or cube. If you don't need all of it, you can boil it down until it has reduced to half its volume, put it into the freezer – I often freeze it in ice-cube trays – then add it to an equal amount of boiling water and use as required.

Put all the ingredients into a large saucepan, cutting them to fit if necessary. Bring slowly to the boil and simmer for 40 minutes. Strain and use as required.

my salad dressing

extra-virgin olive oil	300ml
white wine vinegar	100ml
Dijon mustard	1 tbsp
spring onions	2, very finely chopped
garlic	1 clove, very finely chopped
parsley	1 tsp chopped leaves

Mix all the ingredients together in a bowl. Transfer to a screw-topped jar and shake well. Serve. This will keep for up to 2 weeks, unrefrigerated.

cold beetroot and apple soup

beetroot	500g, uncooked, peeled and grated
onion	1, finely sliced
apple juice	1 litre
lemon	juice of 1
sour cream	150ml
salt and black pepper	to season

Beetroot has a natural high sugar content, making it an excellent source of energy. It also has significant blood-building properties. Combined with health-giving apples, this soup is unusual and refreshing for those hot, exhausting summer days.

Put the beetroot and onion into a food processor with half the apple juice and whizz until smooth. Add the rest of the juice, plus the lemon juice and sour cream. Stir well, season to taste with salt and pepper and chill in the fridge until ready to serve.

vegetable, bean and barley soup

pot barley	45g
carrots	4, finely sliced
turnip	1, chopped
leeks	2, sliced
celery	2 stalks, sliced
onion	1, chopped
tomato purée	1 tbsp
water	1 litre
kidney beans	1 x 400g can, drained and rinsed

An amazing combination of instant and slow-release energy, this typical peasant dish is cheap, filling and nourishing.

Bring the first 7 ingredients to the boil in the water. Simmer for 45 minutes until tender. Add the kidney beans and cook for a further 5 minutes. Ladle into soup bowls and serve immediately.

cabbage soup with potatoes

Savoy cabbage	¼, roughly chopped
potatoes	350g, peeled and cubed
onion	1, large, finely sliced
carrots	2, large
very veggie stock (see recipe, page 97)	1.2 litres
chives	20 stems
dill	3 sprigs
nutmeg	2 pinches, fresh

Top and tail the carrots, peel if not organic and slice. Put the cabbage, potatoes, onion and carrots into a large saucepan. Add the stock and simmer until the potatoes and carrots are tender. Add the chives, dill and nutmeg. Transfer the soup to a blender or food processor and whizz until smooth. Alternatively, use a wand whisk. Ladle into soup bowls and serve.

hauser broth

carrots	125g
celery	3 stalks, finely chopped, with their leaves
spinach or chard	75g finely chopped leaves
water	1.5 litres
runny honey	1 level tbsp
tomato purée	2 tbsp
chives	1 tbsp, finely snipped

Gaylord Hauser was one of the pioneering American naturopaths during the golden era of Hollywood. All the great stars of the 1940s, 1950s and 1960s flocked to see him. He was an extraordinary man, who exuded energy from every pore. He gave me this recipe, which he used in his fasting regimes as an energy booster.

Put the carrots, celery and spinach or chard into a saucepan with the water. Simmer for 30 minutes. Add the tomato purée and honey and cook for a further 5 minutes. Transfer the soup to a blender or food processor and whizz until smooth. Ladle into soup bowls, sprinkle the snipped chives on top and serve.

leek and potato soup

extra-virgin olive oil	4 tbsp
leeks	2, large, trimmed and roughly chopped
potatoes	450g, peeled and cubed
basic chicken stock (see recipe, page 96)	1.2 litres
flat-leaf parsley	4 tbsp finely chopped leaves, plus extra to garnish
live natural yoghurt	500g

This traditional soup is a great source of energy thanks to the carbohydrate in the potatoes. Combined with the protection for the heart and circulation given by the leeks, it's an extremely healthy soup as well. For something really different, use sweet potatoes. Their high betacarotene content provides a huge immune boost.

Heat the oil in a large saucepan and sauté the leeks gently for about 10 minutes. Add the potatoes and continue to cook for about 5 minutes. Pour in the stock and simmer until the potatoes are tender, about 15 minutes. Transfer to a blender or food processor and whizz until smooth. Return to the heat, add the parsley and simmer for 5 minutes. Stir in the yoghurt and garnish with the extra parsley.

For a cold version, strain the mixture after it has been whizzed. Mix in the yoghurt, but omit the chopped parsley and garnish with chopped leaves.

traditional chicken soup

chicken	1 carcass
water	1.2 litres
bouquet garni	1 sachet
bay leaves	3
new potatoes	250g
carrots, parsnips,	450g mixed, cut into
turnips, swede	even-sized cubes
leeks	2, thickly sliced
celery	2 stalks, thickly sliced
Parmesan cheese	4 tbsp, freshly grated

Jewish penicillin may be a joke, but scientific evidence now proves that it really does work. With all the root vegetables, this is a great energy-giver too.

Put the chicken carcass in a large saucepan and pour over the water. Add the bouquet garni and bay leaves and simmer for about 1 hour. Remove the carcass from the pan and fork off any loosened flesh. Halve or quarter the potatoes if large, then add with the rest of the vegetables and simmer until tender, about 30 minutes. Remove and discard the bouquet garni and bay leaves. Ladle into soup bowls and serve sprinkled with the Parmesan cheese.

bread and tomato salad

wholemeal bread	10 medium slices
garlic	4 cloves
extra-virgin olive oil	150ml
plum tomatoes	6, fat, roughly chopped
lemon	juice of 1
mixed soft-leaf herbs	5 tbsp, chopped
black pepper	to season

Nothing could be a quicker, easier or more instant source of energy than this typical dish from southern Spain.

Remove the crusts from the bread and cube. Chop the garlic finely. Heat the oil in a large frying pan, add the bread and garlic and toss until all the oil is absorbed and the bread is just beginning to turn golden. Transfer to a salad bowl, add the tomatoes, lemon juice, herbs and plenty of black pepper. Toss well to serve.

red, white and green coleslaw

carrots	2, grated
cabbage	¼ , white
onion	1, small, finely chopped
sultanas	4 tbsp
live natural yoghurt	200g
extra-virgin olive oil	4 tbsp
cider vinegar	1 tbsp
allspice	1 tsp

Mix the vegetables and sultanas together in a large serving bowl. Whisk the oil, vinegar and allspice together separately and drizzle this dressing over the salad. Mix thoroughly and serve.

spanish salad

tomatoes	500g, roughly chopped
red peppers	2, deseeded and sliced lengthways
green pepper	1, deseeded and sliced lengthways
cucumber	1, medium, peeled, deseeded and cubed
onion	1, large, sweet, white, roughly chopped
parsley	10 sprigs, leaves finely chopped
my salad dressing (see recipe, page 97)	125ml

Just put all the ingredients into a large bowl and toss thoroughly.

tuna and mixed bean salad

tuna	1 x 400g can
beans	1 x 450g can mixed,
red onion	1, large, finely chopped
my salad dressing (see recipe, page 97)	100ml
eggs	2, hard-boiled and quartered
parsley	4 tbsp freshly chopped leaves

This is a perfect lunch if you have a busy afternoon ahead. The beans provide an abundance of instant slow-release energy, and the tuna is an excellent source of easily digested protein to give your brain a boost.

Drain and flake the tuna and drain and rinse the beans. Mix together the fish, beans and onion. Pour over the salad dressing and mix again. Arrange the eggs on top and scatter the parsley over.

tomato and red onion salad

beef tomatoes	4, finely sliced
onions	2, large, finely sliced
my salad dressing (see recipe, page 97)	100ml
basil	½ handful roughly torn leaves

Arrange the tomato and onion slices around the sides of the serving plates. Drizzle the dressing on top and sprinkle with the basil leaves. Serve immediately.

papaya and watercress salad

watercress	2 large bunches, thick stems removed
papaya	1 large, peeled, seeds removed and sliced
beef tomatoes	2, large, sliced
lime	juice of 1
fresh coriander	1 bunch, finely chopped
walnut oil	2 tbsp

An unusual mixture, which tastes as good as it looks. There are energy-stimulating essential oils in the coriander, natural sugars in the tomatoes and papaya and an abundance of energy-boosting protective chemicals in the watercress.

Put the watercress on a large serving plate. Arrange alternate slices of papaya and tomato on top. Mix together the lime juice, coriander and walnut oil and drizzle the dressing on top. Serve immediately.

hummous

chickpeas	1 x 400g can, drained and washed
lemon	juice of 1
garlic	2 cloves, peeled and finely grated
mint	3 large sprigs, roughly torn, and 4 sprigs left whole
extra-virgin olive oil	2 tbsp

Put the first 3 ingredients and the torn mint into a blender or food processor and whizz until blended. Keep the machine running and gradually add the olive oil until the mixture is smooth. Transfer to a serving dish. Garnish with mint sprigs and serve.

guacamole

avocados	2
lemon	juice of 1
live natural yoghurt	100g
tomatoes	1 x 200g can, drained
garlic	3 cloves, very finely chopped
Tabasco sauce	1 tsp

Mash the avodado flesh and mix thoroughly with the rest of the ingredients. Transfer to a serving dish with the avocado stones – this stops the mixture from going brown. Remove the stones before serving.

avocado, tomato and mozzarella salad

avocados	2, cubed
cherry tomatoes	8, halved
mozzarella cheese	1 piece, cubed
chickpeas	1 x 400g can, drained and well rinsed
my salad dressing (see recipe, page 97)	100ml
basil	6 fresh sprigs, leaves removed and roughly torn

Put the first 4 ingredients into a large serving bowl. Pour over the salad dressing and mix well. Scatter the basil leaves on top just before serving.

channel island potato salad

Jersey Royal potatoes	700g
sun-dried tomato paste	3 tbsp
lemon	juice of ½
mixed peppers	2 x 300g jars, drained
feta cheese	110g, cubed
stoned olives	75g, black or green
basil	2 sprigs, leaves roughly torn

Jersey Royal potatoes are unique in their flavour and are suitable for a variety of uses. Any new potatoes will provide energy, but Jerseys are best when available. This terrific energy salad also has lots of immune-boosting vitamin C, cancer-protective lycopene from the tomato paste and calcium and protein from the cheese.

Cook the potatoes in a large saucepan of boiling water. Mix together the sun-dried tomato paste and lemon juice. Drain the potatoes and put them, still warm, into a large serving bowl. Add the peppers, cutting them into fine slivers if too large. Pour on the dressing. When the potatoes are cold, add the feta cheese and olives. Scatter the basil leaves on top and serve.

puddings

spiced baked apples

ground almonds	2 tbsp
raisins	1 tbsp
orange juice	1 tbsp
cooking apples	4, washed, cored and with the bottom 1cm of the core replaced
cloves	4
unsalted butter	50g
brown sugar	1 tbsp
freshly ground nutmeg	4 pinches

The simple addition of ground almonds and raisins adds valuable energy-giving calories and a host of other essential nutrients to this simple dessert.

Preheat the oven to 190°C/375°F/Gas 5. Mix together the almonds, raisins and orange juice. Spoon into the cored cavities of the apples. Top each one with a clove. Use half the butter to grease a large ovenproof dish and the other half to smear over the apple skins. Place the apples in the dish, sprinkle over the sugar and nutmeg and bake in the preheated oven for 25 minutes.

mango and kiwi sorbet

brown caster sugar	225g
rosewater	250ml
kiwi fruit	2, peeled and cube
mango	1, medium, ripe, peeled and cubed
mint	8 leaves, roughly torn
egg white	1

Boil the sugar and rosewater for 1 minute until the sugar is dissolved. Remove from the heat and leave to cool. Put the fruit and mint into a blender or food processor and whizz until smooth. Add the rosewater syrup and egg white and whizz again. Pour into a shallow, freezer-proof container and put into the freezer until almost solid. Take out, mash well with a fork and return to the freezer until solid again. Leave at moderate room temperature for 20 minutes before serving.

orange and mango fool

mangoes	2, ripe, peeled and cubed
orange	juice and grated rind of 1 small
live natural yoghurt	200g

Put all the ingredients into a blender or food processor and whizz until smooth. Spoon into serving bowls, chill then serve.

honeyed plums

red plums	450g, washed but left whole
runny honey	2 tbsp
red wine	4 tbsp
cardamon pods	6
brandy	1 tbsp
fromage frais	200ml

Put the plums, honey, wine and cardamom pods into a large saucepan, cover and simmer until the plums begin to break up, about 8–10 minutes. Add the brandy and heat through for 1 minute. Transfer to serving bowls and serve with the fromage frais.

banana and mango crumble

mango	1, large, cubed
bananas	4, peeled and thickly sliced
lemon	juice and grated rind of 1
soft brown sugar	2 tbsp
muesli	100g, organic
wholemeal breadcrumbs	175g
unsalted butter	100g

Yes, this crumble is made with butter, but there really isn't an alternative, so don't even try to think of one. It provides lots of energy, plus plenty of potassium from the bananas and loads of betacarotene from the mangoes. And it's delicious.

Preheat the oven to 190˚C/375˚F/Gas 5. Mix together the mango, bananas, lemon juice and rind and half the sugar. Pour into a lightly greased pie dish. Mix together the breadcrumbs and 75g of the butter. Add the rest of the sugar and the muesli. Mix thoroughly and pour evenly over the top of the fruit. Dot with the rest of the butter and cook in the preheated oven for 20 minutes.

dried fruit compôte

prunes	110g, stones removed
dried apricots	110g
dried figs	110g
raisins	50g
rosehip teabags	2
runny honey	2 tbsp
cloves	4
live natural yoghurt	300g
lemon	grated zest of 1
cinnamon	1 tsp
flaked almonds	25g

Wash the fruit under cold running water and put into a large bowl with the teabags, honey and cloves. Cover completely with freshly boiled water, stir and leave to cool. Remove the teabags and strain the fruit into 2 bowls. Mix the yoghurt, lemon zest and cinnamon in a separate bowl. Serve the fruit with the yoghurt sauce on top, then sprinkled with the almonds.

index

Answers to anagrams
1 Parliament
2 Clint Eastwood
3 Mental energy
4 Super energy detox
5 Exodus
6 Beefburger
7 Brainstorming

Answers to mental maths
1 112
2 11
3 48
4 6
5 143
6 1000
7 4,777,800

acknowledgements

Three years ago our farmer pal. Malc, asked if he could put four of his Highland cattle in our field for a couple of months. Happily for my wife, Sally, and me, these magnificent long-haired, long-horned and placid animals are still there. They've now been joined by Big Bill, a gorgeous Hereford bull, to whom this series of detox books is dedicated.

Bill is the epitome of health, energy and radiance. He's immensely strong, boundlessly active, and his wonderful mahogany-coloured coat has the feel and texture of the finest silk.

Whether you're reading Super Health Detox, Super Energy Detox or Super Radiance Detox, you could all learn from Bill. He lives in an organic field, where he eats what nature intended for him – natural grasses, wild flowers and herbs – which provide all his essential nutrients. If we all lived a little closer to nature, we'd all be healthier, more energetic and more radiant.

I have to thank Sally for her tireless efforts with the recipes, and everyone at Quadrille for the beautiful design of this book. Special thanks must go to Hilary Mandleberg for her understanding, insight and incredible patience.

picture credits

1 Gettyimages/Peter Nicholson; 2-3 Digital Vision; 4-5 Digital Vision; 14-15 Digital Vision; 17 Gettyimages/Bill Losh; 27 Digital Vision; 29 Digital Vision; 30 Digital Vision; 35 ImageState; 37 Digital Vision; 43 Gettyimages/PBJ Pictures; 44-5 Gettyimages/Steven Rothfeld; 50 Zefa Visual Media UK Ltd/E.Holub; 55 Gettyimages/Dennis O'Clair; 61 Zefa Visual Media UK Ltd/F.Hirdes; 67 Gettyimages/Deborah Jaffe; 68 Digital Vision; 71 Gettyimages/Michael Goldman; 73 Digital Vision; 74 Digital Vision; 78 Digital Vision.

Editorial Director: Jane O'Shea
Consultant Art Director: Françoise Dietrich
Art Editor: Rachel Gibson
Project Editor: Hilary Mandleberg
Production: Nancy Roberts

First published in 2003 by
Quadrille Publishing Limited
Alhambra House
27–31 Charing Cross Road
London WC2H 0LS

Copyright © Text 2003 Michael van Straten
Copyright © Recipes 2003 Sally Pearce
Copyright © Design and layout 2003
Quadrille Publishing Ltd

The rights of Michael van Straten and Sally Pearce to be identified as the authors of this work have been asserted by them in accordance with the Copyright, Design and Patents Act 1988.

British Library Cataloguing-in-Publication Data
A catalogue record for this book is available from the British Library.

ISBN 1 903845 81 5
Printed in Spain